W9-BYR-749

TRANSCEND
FEAR

TRANSCEND
FEAR

A Blueprint for
Mindful Leadership
in Public Health

DR. JOSEPH LADAPO

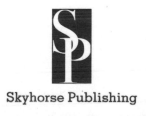

Skyhorse Publishing

Copyright © 2022 by Joseph A. Ladapo

All Rights Reserved. No part of this book may be reproduced in any manner without the express written consent of the publisher, except in the case of brief excerpts in critical reviews or articles. All inquiries should be addressed to Skyhorse Publishing, 307 West 36th Street, 11th Floor, New York, NY 10018.

Skyhorse Publishing books may be purchased in bulk at special discounts for sales promotion, corporate gifts, fund-raising, or educational purposes. Special editions can also be created to specifications. For details, contact the Special Sales Department, Skyhorse Publishing, 307 West 36th Street, 11th Floor, New York, NY 10018 or info@skyhorsepublishing.com.

Skyhorse® and Skyhorse Publishing® are registered trademarks of Skyhorse Publishing, Inc.®, a Delaware corporation.

Visit our website at www.skyhorsepublishing.com.

10 9 8 7 6 5 4 3 2 1

Library of Congress Cataloging-in-Publication Data is available on file.

ISBN: 978-1-5107-7471-1
eBook ISBN: 978-1-5107-7472-8

Cover design by Brian Peterson

Printed in the United States of America

To Brianna, my light and heart.
To Eric, Jack, and Max. Mom and Dad love you always.

Contents

Foreword

by Robert F. Kennedy Jr.

Iatrarchy—meaning government by physicians—is a little-known term, perhaps because historical experiments with it have been catastrophic. The medical profession has not proven itself an energetic defender of democratic institutions or civil rights. Virtually every doctor in Germany took lead roles in the Third Reich's project to eliminate mental defectives, homosexuals, handicapped citizens, and Jews. So many hundreds of German physicians participated in Hitler's worst atrocities—including managing mass murder and unspeakable experiments at the death camps—that the Allies had to stage separate "Medical Trials" at Nuremberg. Not a single prominent German doctor or medical association raised their voice in opposition to these projects.

So it's unsurprising that, instead of demanding blue-ribbon safety science and encouraging honest, open, and responsible debate on the science, the badly compromised and newly empowered government health officials charged with managing the COVID-19 pandemic response collaborated with mainstream and social media to shut down discussion on key public health and civil rights questions.

They silenced and excommunicated heretics who refused to genuflect to Pharma and treat unquestioning faith in economically devastating lockdowns, catastrophic school closures, and zero-liability, shoddily tested, experimental vaccines as religious duty.

Our current iatrarchy's rubric of "scientific consensus" is the contemporary iteration of the Spanish Inquisition. It is a fabricated dogma constructed by this corrupt cast of physician technocrats and their media collaborators to legitimize their claims to dangerous new powers.

The high priests of the modern Inquisition are Big Pharma's network and cable news gasbags who preach rigid obedience to official diktats including lockdowns, social distancing, and the moral rectitude of donning masks despite the absence of peer-reviewed science that convincingly shows that masks prevent COVID-19 transmission. The need for this sort of proof is gratuitous.

They counsel us to, instead, "trust the experts." Such advice is both antidemocratic and antiscience. Science is dynamic. "Experts" frequently differ on scientific questions, and their opinions can vary in accordance with and demands of politics, power, and financial self-interest. Nearly every lawsuit I have ever brought pitted highly credentialed experts from opposite sides against each other, with all of them swearing under oath to diametrically antithetical positions based on the same set of facts. *Science is disagreement; the notion of scientific consensus is oxymoronic.*

Instead of citing scientific studies to justify mandates for masks, lockdowns, and vaccines, our medical rulers cite WHO, CDC, FDA, and NIH-captive agencies that are groveling sock puppets to the industries they regulate. Multiple federal and international investigations have documented the financial entanglements with pharmaceutical companies that have made these regulators cesspools of corruption.

In 2020, led by Bill Gates, Silicon Valley applauded from the sidelines as powerful medical charlatans—applying the most pessimistic projections from discredited modeling and easily manipulated PCR testing, and a menu of new protocols for coroners that appeared intended to inflate reporting of COVID-19 deaths—fanned pandemic panic and confined the world's population under house arrest.

In America, their quarantine predictably shattered the nation's once-booming economic engine, putting 58 million Americans out of work and *permanently bankrupting over 100,000 small businesses,*

including 41,000 Black-owned businesses, some of which took three gener-
ations of investment to build. These policies have also set into motion
the inevitable dismantling of the social safety net that nurtured America's envied middle class. Government officials have already begun
liquidating the 100-year legacies of the New Deal, the New Frontier,
the Great Society, and Obamacare to pay the accumulated quarantine
debts. Say good-bye to school lunches, healthcare, WIC, Medicaid,
Medicare, University scholarships, and more.

Their government/industry collaboration will use this system to
manage the rage when Americans finally wake up to the fact that this
outlaw gang has stolen our democracy, civil rights, country, and way of
life—while we huddled in orchestrated fear from a flu-like illness.

A consummate insider, the former White House Chief of Staff Rahm
Emmanuel is known for his admonition that vested power structures
should "never let a serious crisis to go to waste." But this tread-worn
strategy—to use crisis to inflame the public terror that paves the road
to dictatorial power—has served as the central strategy of totalitarian
systems for the millennia.

The methodology is, in fact, formulaic, as Hiller's Luftwaffe com-
mander, Hermann Göring, explained during the Nazi war crimes trials
at Nuremberg: "It is always a simple matter to drag the people along
whether it is a democracy, a fascist dictatorship, or a parliament, or a
communist dictatorship. Voice or no voice, the people can always be
brought to the bidding of the leaders. That is easy. All you have to do is
tell them they are being attacked, and denounce the pacifists for lack of
patriotism, and exposing the country to greater danger. It works the same
in any country."

Demagogues must weaponize fear to justify their demands for blind
obedience and to win public acquiescence for the demolition of civil and
economic rights. Of course, the first casualty must always be freedom of
speech. In including free speech in the First Amendment of the Constitution, James Madison argued that all our other liberties depend on this
right. Any government that can hide its mischief has license to commit
atrocities.

As soon as they get hold of the levers of authority, tyrants impose Orwellian censorship and begin gaslighting dissenters. But ultimately, they seek to abolish all forms of creative thinking and self-expression. They burn books; destroy art; kill writers, poets, and intellectuals; outlaw gatherings; and, at their worst, force oppressed minorities to wear masks that atomize any sense of community or solidarity and prevent the subtle, eloquent nonverbal communication for which God and evolution have equipped humans with 42 facial muscles. The most savage Middle Eastern theocracies mandate masks for women, whose legal status—not coincidentally—is as chattels.

The free flow of information and self-expression are oxygen and sunlight for representative democracy, which functions best with policies annealed in the boiling cauldron of public debate. It is axiomatic that without free speech, democracy withers.

Predictably, our other constitutional guarantees lined up behind free speech at the gibbet. The imposition of censorship has masked this systematic demolition of our Constitution, including attacks on our freedoms of assembly (through social distancing and lockdown rules), worship (including abolishing religious exemptions and closing churches, while liquor stores remain open as "essential service"), private property (the right to operate a business), due process (including the imposition of far-reaching restrictions against freedoms of movement, education, and association without rulemaking, public hearings, or economic and environmental impact statements), in addition to the Seventh Amendment right to jury trials (in cases of vaccine injuries caused by corporate negligence), our rights to privacy and against illegal searches and seizures (warrantless tracking and tracing), and our right to have governments that don't spy on us or retain our information for mischievous purposes.

The persecution of scientists and doctors who dare to challenge contemporary orthodoxies is not a new phenomenon. As he left the Roman Inquisition tribunal before which he repudiated his theory that the Earth—the immovable center of the Universe according to contemporary orthodoxy—revolves around the sun, Galileo whispered, "And yet, it moves." Had he not recanted, his life would be forfeited.

Nor did the silencing of scientists and doctors not take a rest after Galileo: it has always been, and remains today, an occupational hazard. Henrik Ibsen's 1882 play, *An Enemy of the People,* is a parable for the pitfall of scientific integrity. Ibsen tells the story of a doctor in southern Norway who discovers that his town's popular and lucrative public baths were actually sickening the visitors who flocked to them for rejuvenation. Discharges from local tanneries had infected the spas with lethal bacteria. When the doctor goes public with the information, local merchants, joined by government officials, their allies in the "liberal-minded independent press," and other financially interested parties move to muzzle him. The medical establishment pulls his medical license, the townsfolk vilify and brand him "an enemy of the people."

Ibsen's fictional doctor experienced what social scientists call the "Semmelweis reflex." This term describes the knee-jerk revulsion with which the press, the medical and scientific community, and allied financial interests greet new scientific evidence that contradicts an established scientific paradigm. The reflex can be particularly fierce in cases where new scientific information suggests that established medical practices are actually harming public health.

The real-life plight of Ignaz Semmelweis, a Hungarian physician, inspired the term and Ibsen's play. In 1847, Dr. Semmelweis was an assistant professor at Vienna's General Hospital maternity clinic, where around 10 percent of women died from puerperal "birth bed" fever. Based on his pet theory that cleanliness could mitigate transmission of disease-causing "particles," Semmelweis introduced the practice of mandatory hand washing for interns between performing autopsies and delivering babies. The rate of fatal puerperal fever immediately dropped to around 1 percent. Semmelweis published these findings.

Rather than building a statue to Semmelweis, the medical community, unwilling to admit culpability in the injury of so many patients, expelled the doctor from the medical profession. His former colleagues tricked Dr. Semmelweis into visiting a mental institution in 1865, then committed him against his will. Semmelweis died mysteriously two weeks later. A decade afterward, Louis Pasteur's germ theory and Joseph Lister's work on hospital sanitation vindicated Semmelweis's ideas.

We like to think of Galileo's struggles as the quaint artifact of a dark, ignorant, and tyrannical era where individuals challenged government-anointed superstitions only at grave personal risk. The COVID-19 pandemic—and the disastrous, corrupt, fear-induced management of it by public health officials—shows that stubborn orthodoxies anointed by pharmaceutical companies and corrupt government regulators to protect power and profits remain a dominant force in science and politics.

From his writings in the *Wall Street Journal* to his speech in front of the Supreme Court to his role as the surgeon general of Florida, Dr. Joseph Ladapo has shown tremendous courage in the face of extraordinary resistance on the part of the Big Pharma, corrupt government regulators, and his own colleagues.

For Dr. Ladapo—as for so many others—the pandemic has served as a wake-up call. A successful career in medicine had led him to expect from the medical and scientific community a certain level of rational thinking. Years spent as a clinician and researcher had taught him the value of a logical analysis of the available data, an open-minded approach to solving crises, and a decision-making framework aimed at helping rather than harming. The pandemic exposed just the opposite. Suddenly, physicians, researchers, and public health leaders at the highest levels were promoting policy ideas that had no basis in science or in the available data. These policies—lockdowns, masks, unproven vaccines—were grounded, instead, in fear and pushed by corrupt political characters and pharmaceutical interests. They would prove devastating for untold millions of people.

With clarity and bravery, Dr. Ladapo wrote about these issues in the *Wall Street Journal* from the beginning of the pandemic. His compassion and intelligence touched many readers who felt they—not the CDC, the FDA, or the NIH—knew what was best for their children and their families. Unsurprisingly, he was castigated by his colleagues in the medical community, and attempts to discredit him proliferated in all corners of the media.

He was—and remains—steadfast in his principles. As the surgeon general of Florida, his voice has become one of the most important in the fight for freedom over fear, personal rights over government mandates, and science-based public health policy over ideologically driven rulemaking.

It's a bad omen for democracy when citizens can no longer conduct civil, informed debates about critical policies that impact the vitality of our economy, public health, personal freedoms, and constitutional rights. Censorship is violence, and this systematic muzzling of debate—which proponents justify as a measure to curtail dangerous polarization—is actually fueling the polarization and extremism that the autocrats use to clamp down with evermore draconian controls.

Valery Legasov, the courageous Russian physicist who braved censor, torture, and threats on his life by the KGB to reveal to the world the true cause of the Chernobyl disaster, was quoted as saying: "To be a scientist is to be naive. We are so focused on our search for the truth, we fail to consider how few actually want us to find it. But it is always there, whether we can see it or not, whether we choose to or not. The truth doesn't care about our needs or our wants. It doesn't care about our governments, our ideologies, our religions. It will lie in wait for all time."

Science, at its best, is a search for existential truth. Sometimes, however, those truths threaten powerful economic paradigms. Both science and democracy rely on the free flow of accurate information. Greedy corporations and captive government regulators have consistently shown themselves willing to twist, distort, falsify, and corrupt science, hide information, and censor open debate to protect personal power and corporate profits. Censorship is the fatal enemy of both democracy and public health.

If we are to continue to enjoy democracy and protect our children from the forces that seek to commoditize humanity, then we need courageous scientists, like Joseph Ladapo, who are willing to search for that existential truth and speak truth to power, even at a personal cost.

CHAPTER 1

Getting the Call

In late August 2021, I received an unexpected phone call. About a week earlier, I had received an email from Florida Governor Ron DeSantis's chief of staff, Adrian Lukis. However, we had just moved into a new house, were busy trying to sort out childcare and schooling for our three kids, and I was juggling three large clinical studies in my job as a professor at UCLA. So, unbeknownst to me, the email I wrote in response sat unsent in my Draft messages folder.

After not hearing from the governor's office for a few days, I took another look at my email and noticed the unsent reply. I remember thinking, *Oh, not again,* and forwarding the message, along with an apology for the delay and a request that they contact me by phone in the future. I hated to drop the ball with important messages, and I had learned to accept the fact that I would never be as organized as my wife, Brianna, so I had better take extra steps to make communications foolproof.

When we finally connected on the phone, Adrian started the conversation by telling me who he was and explaining that he understood I was on the other side of the country, that my family was settled in California, and that I was a tenured researcher and doctor at UCLA. But, he said, they were looking for a new surgeon general in Florida, and if I was interested...

I remember thinking that his pitch had an air of defeat to it, as if he expected me to say no and didn't think I would possibly uproot my family—or my career. Truthfully, I thought he was right, but I said, "Let me talk to my wife."

Brianna is the family's spiritual and emotional heart. She has made this journey possible, and I would not be where I am today without her. She has also nurtured our kids emotionally and spiritually and taught me how to do the same. Our three boys are amazing, unique, beautiful, joyful, and powerful little guys, and none of us would be who we are without her.

At the time of the phone call, Los Angeles was still under lockdown. Though not quite as intense as at the beginning of the pandemic, it was still impossible to go most places without encountering one type of pandemic restriction or another, so I was working from home that day. I remember taking the call on my way to the mailbox next to the driveway. Brianna was out. When she got home, as she was walking into the kitchen, I said, "Honey, I got a call from Governor DeSantis's office."

She snapped around. "Really?"

"Yeah, they want me to consider being the surgeon general."

She looked as though she'd been waiting to hear a message and it had finally arrived. She didn't hesitate. "You should do it," she said.

It was not how I expected the conversation to go. Our kids, who were eight, four, and two at that point, were getting used to the homeschooling routine we were putting together for them with other like-minded parents. The Los Angeles Unified School District had reopened, but they required masks, social distancing, and COVID testing, all of which my wife and I agreed created a needlessly harmful environment for our two older boys, who were eligible for enrollment. It was clear from the highest-quality data that the mandates would not actually benefit children and that the school district was taking a politically driven approach to bringing children back to in-person learning—so we refused to participate.

Additionally, we had just moved out of our condo and into a new house with a backyard less than two weeks earlier. Brianna had planted a garden, we had made friends in the neighborhood, and we were freshly unpacked and settling in. I was shocked when, almost without thinking, she told me to do it—to take the job in Florida.

She said, "That's the call. That's what I've been waiting for."

Prior to the pandemic, my relationship with UCLA had been very good. But by late summer 2021, as a result of the stances I had taken on COVID-19 policies, things had deteriorated into something resembling a bad marriage.

I was annoyed about it, but Brianna was completely out of patience. She had long felt I'd outgrown UCLA and saw the institution as a pandering oppressor of free speech and critical thought. My feeling was that I was a tenured professor, my research and patient care were going well, and even though it wasn't a great environment—with some of my colleagues calling for my dismissal and revocation of my medical license because I expressed disagreement with their politicization of the pandemic—I was performing well at my job, so there was little official action they could take against me.

But Brianna was clear: that was the call.

I called Adrian back and said I was interested.

The next day, I had a pleasant interview with Governor DeSantis. He'd become aware of me through my writings in the *Wall Street Journal*, and through a few doctors and researchers I'd been in touch with throughout the pandemic on policy and lockdown issues. I found out later that the governor had appreciated the fact that the core aspects of my message had remained the same from the very beginning.

I got another call from Adrian the next day.

"Governor DeSantis wants to offer you the job," he said.

From that point on, my wife and I started working out how we were going to move our lives from Los Angeles to Florida. That first night, after we put the kids to bed, we looked at a map of Florida and started learning more about different cities. "I can't live in Tallahassee," Brianna said. "But I could live in Tampa."

She just didn't think Tallahassee was vibrant enough for our family to thrive there, and Brianna's intuition and instinct have always served as a guiding light for our family. I was relieved when I spoke with Adrian the next day and he said he didn't think commuting would be a problem. Then it was just a matter of details.

But I also had to figure out what to do in relation to UCLA and my academic work as a clinical researcher. I had a few options.

I brought the news to my boss, Carol Mangione, who was my division chief at UCLA. Before the pandemic, we'd had a warm and collegial relationship, and I truly admired her. She was incisive, creative, extraordinarily capable, and formidable. And early on, she was supportive—proud even—of the fact that one of her faculty members was publishing articles in the *Wall Street Journal*, a rarity in academia.

But as the pandemic climate became more overtly political, and the "right" answers and "correct" positions became more loudly and monotonously dictated by authorities, public health officials, and universities, she found herself forced to reconcile her feelings about me with her opposition to my ideas. It was not an easy position for her.

The tension between us grew with each newly published article and each television interview invitation. She employed multiple strategies to either deter me from expressing my opinion or make the process more burdensome. Some of the things she did were clearly out of line with UCLA's policies on academic freedom. Once, she suggested to me that I was violating the Hippocratic Oath to do no harm, to which I gently explained how the lockdown policies supported by many public officials—such as keeping children out of school—were, in fact, very harmful to health.

But she was in a difficult position. She later told me that people were calling her "weak" because she hadn't fired me, which she could not have done anyway without inviting a lawsuit, considering that I was a high-performing member of the department. More than once, she explained to me that a substantial part of her workday was spent dealing with complaints about my writings, including from donors to UCLA.

When I told her that I had been offered the position of surgeon general of the state of Florida, her initial reaction was shock. It was discernible over the phone, as her voice changed and became punctuated with disorientation. As the news settled in, we discussed a few options in relation to UCLA. One idea we discussed was to take a leave of absence. A second idea was to try and continue both positions, although this seemed logistically infeasible and could introduce conflicts of interest. Fortunately, she contacted the chair of the Department of Medicine, Dr. Alan Fogelman.

To my surprise, Dr. Fogelman told me he enjoyed reading my articles and extended a warm congratulations on the job offer. Invaluably, he advised me to seek out a tenured faculty position in Florida. Since I was a tenured faculty member at UCLA, one of the most prestigious research universities in the country, he felt that a tenured position in Florida would not only be wise, but appropriate.

His warmth and appreciation of the gravity of the announcement helped reorient my immediate boss, Dr. Mangione, and she suddenly snapped into a mode of being helpful. She offered to write a letter of support for an application to the University of Florida.

With that settled, we then had to find a place to live. I mentioned to a friend, Bruce, who lived in the Tampa area that we were trying to figure out where to live and looking at Hillsborough County. He said, "Don't go to Hillsborough County. They are one of the counties defying the governor's order to not mask kids in school. Move to Pinellas County. It's less crazy there, more in touch with reality." So we did just that.

In a whirlwind two weeks, we packed and wrapped up our affairs in California so we could get to Florida and start our lives there. We especially wanted to get the kids settled and back in school as soon as possible.

On Friday, September 18, I received the offer letter from the University of Florida, on Sunday I flew to Tallahassee, and on Monday, Governor DeSantis made the announcement that he was appointing me to the role of surgeon general of Florida.

"I am pleased to announce that Dr. Joseph Ladapo will lead the Florida Department of Health as our state's next surgeon general. Dr. Ladapo comes to us by way of the David Geffen School of Medicine at UCLA with a superb background. He has had both a remarkable academic and medical career with a strong emphasis in health policy research. Dr. Ladapo will bring great leadership to the Department of Health."

That morning, I told the governor that, during the press conference, I specifically wanted to discuss rejecting fear, basing decisions on data rather than politics, and emphasizing preventive and overall health. To my surprise and delight, he told me to go for it without even a moment's hesitation. I was impressed. "I am honored to have been chosen by Governor DeSantis to serve as Florida's next surgeon general," I said. "We must make health policy decisions rooted in data and not in fear. From California, I have observed the different approaches taken by governors across the country, and I have been impressed by Governor DeSantis's leadership and determination to ensure that Floridians are afforded all opportunities to maintain their health and wellness, while preserving their freedoms as Americans. It is a privilege to join his team and serve the people of Florida."

We issued a new emergency rule ending mandatory quarantines for healthy students exposed to people with COVID-19 that very day.

It was a simple message, but it sounded very alien at the time.

I had to fly back to Los Angeles soon after, but a few days later my wife, our three kids, and I got on a plane to Tampa, checked into an Airbnb late that night, and embarked on the next chapter of our lives.

CHAPTER 2

Growing Up

I was born in Nigeria. My parents, looking for a better life for themselves and their three kids, came to the United States when I was about five years old. We settled first in Baton Rouge, Louisiana, where my dad was a graduate student at Louisiana State University, and then in Athens, Georgia. Under an extremely kind supervisor at the University of Georgia, my father earned his PhD in microbiology. My mother earned a bachelor's degree in business there, as well.

My parents were students and didn't have much money, so we lived in university housing in Louisiana and Georgia. But it was a great environment for childhood fun, especially in Georgia, because the apartments were sprawling with great sidewalks for bike riding and great hills for grass sledding. I remember passing weekends and summer days running around, playing kickball and other games with kids in the neighborhood.

When we moved to Athens, Georgia, our parents enrolled us in St. Joseph's Catholic School. The principal was a woman named Sister Helen Gilroy, with whom I'm still in touch to this day. Despite the fact that I was, by and large, a good student, I was in her office many, many times. I'd get into trouble—nothing terrible—but I often couldn't sit still or stop goofing off in class. I didn't realize it at the time, but attention seeking was my subconscious motivation. Fortunately, that was clear to Sister Helen.

My father was a domineering force in the family. My mother, by nature, was gentle and nurturing, but it was my father who set the tone for all of us. He grew up under very challenging circumstances in Nigeria—unaffectionate, rigid, and full of unfortunate suffering. Corporal punishment was common for him growing up and was an accepted part of the culture in his community.

His behavior and approach to the world and relating to others, including his wife and kids, was shaped—defined, even—by the trauma he experienced as a child. He did the best he could, but with a childhood like his and no opportunities to address those injuries and heal, he—like most people harboring unhealed trauma—was destined to leave emotional wreckage in his wake when he married and had children. Unsurprisingly, my father believed heavily in corporal punishment himself, and I received the most of it among my siblings.

Sometimes I think about how different our kids' childhood is from my own, and it almost takes my breath away. They are enveloped in safety, tons of affection, and the freedom to *be*, and Brianna and I have a warm, squishy emotional connection with each of the little guys.

After my parents earned their degrees, we moved to North Carolina, where I spent my junior and senior years of high school at the North Carolina School of Science and Math. My parents pushed my siblings and me to do well academically, and the good grades I earned as a result of that pressure opened a lot of doors for me.

Growing up, I felt my childhood was a happy one. And while I was a joyous kid by nature, as I look back now, I see clearly that I was emotionally deadened. The amplitude of my emotional capacity was a fraction of what it would have been had I been emotionally healthy. At the time, I truly didn't know; I thought everything was fine. But it was far from fine, and the numbness I experienced was rooted back in Nigeria.

For as long as I can remember, I've had vivid memories of being sexually abused by a babysitter in Nigeria as a young child. My guess is she herself had been sexually abused in her own childhood.

I was probably about four years old—old enough to recognize that what she was doing wasn't right, but too young to know what to do about it, or to have any sense of how to talk to someone about it. It was clearly wrong, but I was so young when it happened, I had no way of processing the experience. She broke my boundaries, and it profoundly affected who I grew to be.

I don't have many memories from my early childhood—but this one is vivid. For years, I thought it had not affected me. I felt that even though I remembered it, it didn't matter. I was fine. It wasn't until I worked through it decades later that I realized I had simply become numb to the experience. In the moment, I was terrified and overwhelmed, and the shattering of my boundaries deadened my ability to create authentic emotional connections with other people.

Sexual predators are among us, and they unfortunately often have an uncanny sense of which kids are good targets. Kids who are less connected with their families, or who have low self-esteem or a weak sense of personal boundaries, are some of the most likely to be preyed upon. As I would later learn, broken boundaries made me a target for sexual predators later in life.

There were predators at my boarding school. The two I remember are a soccer coach who had been a suspected or convicted sex offender in the Midwest and was accused of sexually abusing at least one of the students on our soccer team, and a guy named Emmanuel, who was a supervisor in one of the dormitories.

Emmanuel was in his late twenties or early thirties. On weekends, he would invite boys over to his apartment after curfew, something that was technically against the rules. But at that age, kids think they're cool when they receive that type of invitation. He often played pornographic movies and offered alcohol. I went a few times and remember thinking that the circumstances were strange but interesting.

During my freshman year of college, he invited me to a strip club and offered to give me a massage in a hotel room beforehand. At the time, the encounters seemed benign, but I eventually was able to see them for exactly what they were—a predator's attempts to groom and molest teenagers. And I am sure he picked up on my own emotional disconnection from other people as a sign that I might be vulnerable to his attempts to enroll me in his fantasies. Fortunately, he was unsuccessful with me, though I have no doubt that he was successful with other students.

After high school, I went to Wake Forest University on an academic scholarship. I became a decathlete and cocaptain of the track and field team. I had a successful athletic career and was particularly competitive in the long jump and high hurdles, ranking in the top 10 of our school records in these events, decathlon, and the 4 x 100-meter sprint relay. When I didn't have to be up early for a weekend track and field workout, I joined other students at fraternity parties and hung out with friends. And I did well in my academic courses.

But outside of the classroom and off the track, I was also feeding a growing interest in policy decisions. In particular, I was interested in understanding why people have different perspectives and how those perspectives inform their opinions and outlook. It was this interest that led to me study questions of policy, first as a hobby at Wake Forest University and later at the John F. Kennedy School of Government while I was in medical school at Harvard University.

I had always liked science, but more than that, I liked the idea of a career that would allow me to be a scientist while being of service to other people. Like many immigrants, my parents encouraged us to pursue an advanced professional degree. I applied to several medical schools and felt incredibly lucky to be accepted into Harvard. Of all the schools to which I was admitted, I enjoyed my visit there most. My mom, dad, and I hit the road with directions printed out from MapQuest and made our way to Boston in the summer of 2000.

Brianna flew into my life out of nowhere.

I met her during the summer after my first year at the Kennedy School of Government. I was a student in their Master in Public Policy program, which I started after my third year of medical school. In the first summer of the program, a friend of mine told me she was going to be in St. Croix to work on a project. I didn't have much money, but the beautiful, clear water of the Caribbean had spoken to me for as long as I could remember. As long as I could stay with her, I could afford to go. So I went. It was incredible. I went scuba diving for the first time, snorkeling, and kayaking. I would go on five- or six-mile runs around the island, taking in its beauty and personality. The week was wonderful.

On the way back, I had a connecting flight in San Juan, Puerto Rico. I got on the flight, and one row in front of me, to my right, was a cute girl. I made some small talk with her, asked her some questions, and we ended up talking the entire flight. She had been in St. Thomas with some friends and was headed back to San Diego, where she had her own business writing commercials for companies and doing other creative work.

Hurricane Charlie disrupted connecting flights, so we were separated in Newark, as passengers scrambled to find a way home. Even though I thought I would never see her again, I reflected on the fact that we had a really nice conversation on the plane, and I tracked her down in the airport amid the chaos. We exchanged phone numbers. Thank goodness!

A game of phone tag ensued over the next six months or so, but eventually, we started talking more regularly. As winter rolled into spring, and spring rolled into another summer, we found ourselves having conversations that would last four, six, and even eight hours. On several occasions, we talked so far into the night that I saw the sun rise from my apartment as night broke into day.

I did not know it at the time, but I was falling in love with Brianna over the phone. This was especially divine since we were falling in love with each other's hearts and minds without the added complications of a physical romantic relationship. I was not emotionally well enough to have a healthy physical relationship. And I would have likely pursued just that had Brianna lived in Boston. Somehow Brianna snuck into my heart through a backdoor that God had left unlocked.

Eventually she came to visit, and I remember sitting on the couch with her, watching a movie—*Hotel Rwanda*—feeling absolutely enveloped in a warm blanket of love and affection. I will never forget how content, how secure, how warmly held I felt that night. I'd never felt anything like that before. I kissed her on that visit, but by that point I'd already fallen in love with her.

But as love opened up my heart, it also opened doors to the rooms that hid my emotional and spiritual injuries. It brought to the surface my disconnection from other people and forced me to reconcile that disconnection with the deep connection I now had with Brianna. It brought to the surface the learned belief system that my family—mom, dad, brother, and sister—and their needs came first, no matter what these needs meant for the fortunes of other people. And most profoundly, it brought to the surface a child within me that was stuck in time, frozen by an experience when my boundaries were broken, traumatized by the introduction of a sexual energy that was beyond my capacity to process.

As one of many consequences of the sexual abuse I experienced, I was crippled, intimidated, and terrified by the thought of any prior romantic relationships Brianna had. The part of me that was frozen in time was determined to protect me from reexperiencing its trauma and annihilation—which meant protecting me from her.

When any thought of Brianna potentially being intimate in past relationships with another person came to my mind, this child within me sprang up. As it arrived on the scene, my vision became fuzzy, as if my eyes were looking through a thin, cloudy film. My spirit became groggy and burdened and slow. Unbeknownst to me at the time, I was being transported back to that traumatic experience. I would lose my executive function and ability to make decisions as an adult. I was in a childlike state. I was incapable of answering questions as simple as "which toppings do you want on your pizza?" or "Should I take a taxi or bus to campus?" because I could not access my adult desires or executive planning functions.

Like any unresolved trauma, it was profoundly destructive to my relationship with Brianna. And that was the point—to destroy—because a part of me was threatened by her and by sexuality. It also was why my prior relationships with women were never truly emotionally intimate; there was a boulder in the way determined to protect me.

From this state of being trapped in the past, salvation in the present could only be achieved by putting my mind and attention completely on my love for Brianna and saying the words to myself, under my breath, "I love you." I would repeat the words over and over and put my mind and attention fully on her, and eventually, sometimes after minutes, sometimes after hours, I reentered our love relationship, returned to my present adult self, and was transported back to reality. Usually, that meant it was time to repair whatever damage I had caused our relationship while my inner child was in charge and address whatever issues I couldn't tackle when I was without my executive function and adult decision-making abilities.

This problem was profound in terms of its effect on me, and while I can describe the dynamics clearly now, it was debilitating and far beyond my ability to comprehend at the time. And it was very destructive to my relationship with Brianna. My adult self wanted to live in the squishy comfort and security of that evening on the couch forever, while the child in me wanted to destroy an existential threat. I had never experienced anything like this before and had no idea such an experience even existed.

But as I would later learn, this experience was the first step in my journey toward freedom from fear. When the babysitter broke my boundaries as a child, it filled me with terror and encased my heart in a layer that crippled my ability to authentically connect emotionally with other people. Now, something that should never have been possible—falling in love—happened, and it decimated the conscious and subconscious false beliefs that directed my life.

Great inner struggle was ignited: a struggle between loving Brianna and feeling deeply threatened by her, a struggle between loving my family—who had always been first in my life—and realizing that my heart and soul had now declared that she was first, a struggle between experiencing love and living in a deadened state of emotion. I was on a spiritual and emotional roller coaster.

Fortunately, Brianna had incredible emotional capacity and emotional wisdom, and it was enough to carry us both through the journey. She helped me continuously but also knew that I would need someone to speak with, someone with whom I could share everything, including things that I could not share with her.

She helped me find a therapist, a man who was perfect for a person as untrusting as I was. He was kind, gentle, wise, and nonjudgmental. Most of our time was spent discussing how I felt when I was trapped in time and felt like a little boy, my feelings of being eviscerated and destroyed when issues of sex came up (it would be a while before we peeled away enough layers to uncover this, but we eventually did), and my relationship with my family, especially my dad. In retrospect, it is clear to me now that he was helping me remove, brick by brick, the defensive walls I had built around my heart and upon which I had rigidly framed my consciousness.

Though that therapist helped me tremendously and allowed me to better function and to rescue myself when a thought about sex teleported me back to a childlike state, my struggles were still deep. The problems they created for Brianna and me were omnipresent, and the brick walls stretched as high as skyscrapers.

This meant unyielding pain for Brianna over the years, which was exacerbated when we had kids, and new doors holding other hidden emotional burdens were abruptly forced open. Brianna suffered, and I hated causing her pain but did not have enough mastery of myself and my emotions to prevent it. Her suffering and our struggle eventually led her to find Christopher Maher, a former Navy SEAL who had helped heal many people suffering from trauma. At the end of her rope, she insisted that I see him. And thank the Lord I listened, because after working with him, I finally became truly free.

CHAPTER 3

Beginning My Career

While I was pursuing my medical degree at Harvard Medical School, I was also taking classes at Harvard's John F. Kennedy School of Government. My first year—2003 to 2004—was an election year, and the school was teeming with famous politicians, media leaders, and other business and policy leaders who held seminars and spoke with students. It was an extraordinary experience.

It was at the Kennedy School that I was first introduced to the field of economic theory. I especially benefited from a class taught by Dr. Richard Zeckhauser, a brilliant and eminent economist. Through his class and my other training, I studied analytic frameworks for decision making under uncertainty.

The class materials resonated with me at the deepest levels, and I saw their immediate value to health policy and medical decision making. But I knew that more in-depth study was needed to achieve mastery. In pursuit of this goal, I decided to apply to the PhD Program in Health Policy at Harvard.

In the PhD program, I focused on decision sciences and continued course work in economics and statistics. Decision sciences was a field that focused on optimizing decisions by characterizing the risks, benefits, and trade-offs associated with different choices. While I had a natural affinity for the quantitative methods that formed the foundation of decision sciences, I had no idea how much this training would prove useful during the COVID-19 pandemic. My thesis focused on cardio-vascular disease and evaluation of emerging technologies for diagnosis and management.

Eight years after arriving in Boston, I graduated from medical school and my PhD program. I went on to start my residency in internal medi-cine at the Beth Israel Deaconess Medical Center in Boston. After train-ing there, I sought a faculty position as a clinician researcher and received job offers from Johns Hopkins, UCLA, Columbia, and NYU.

NYU offered a promising environment for mentorship and felt like a place where I could thrive and develop. Brianna and I made the move from Cambridge the day I finished my residency. The movers came that morning, Brianna went ahead to New York, and I caught the bus later that day after seeing my last patient in Boston.

At NYU, my career as a physician scientist began auspiciously. I received a grant from the National Institutes of Health to study diag-nosis and management of cardiovascular disease in the beginning of my second year. Becoming an NIH-funded researcher was an important threshold to cross, and the projects allowed me to build further expertise in survey research, epidemiology, and decision analysis. It was an import-ant milestone in my early career.

I received my second grant, for a clinical trial of smoking cessation strategies in hospitalized patients, from the Robert Wood Johnson Foun-dation. This was the first of several clinical trials I would eventually lead. In addition to the value that comes from answering important clinical questions, clinical trials taught me more about the regulatory aspects of clinical science, how to overcome challenges in running and sustaining clinical trials, and how to effectively work with diverse hospital systems in pursuit of a scientific goal.

The interventions I tested in this trial and in future trials were in the field of behavioral economics, a field that aims to better understand human behavior by merging concepts from conventional economics with intuition and insights about how people make decisions. My spe-cific interest in this area was based on the fact that people often express a desire to make healthy changes to their life habits but frequently are unsuccessful translating these desires into action. I aimed to use strategies from behavioral economics and financial incentives to help increase how likely people were to make the changes they wanted to make. My research also earned me the *Annals of Internal Medicine* Junior Investigator Award.

When I wasn't working on research, I was taking care of patients at the NYU Langone Medical Center as a hospitalist physician. All in all, I was a good example of a guy who appeared to have it all together on the outside but was truly a wreck on the inside, experiencing fearfulness about my job, my prospects for success, and, increasingly, Brianna's health challenges related to her migraines.

Brianna and I were enjoying the city and planning our lives together. When we decided to have kids, Brianna had to stop taking a preventive medication she had been using to manage chronic migraines, from which she'd suffered since she was a little girl. Very quickly, her migraines worsened.

Suddenly, she was having an incredibly rough time, suffering so profoundly that she was hospitalized multiple times for management of intractable migraines. Frequent migraines and crippling pain meant that she was forced to spend many days in bed, unable to fully participate in life.

Meanwhile, my limited ability to manage stress put me into a state of overwhelm, and I felt intensely stressed by the challenges she was dealing with, the calls to emergency medical services for ambulances when she was too incapacitated to travel to the emergency department, and the frequent interactions with medical doctors and nurses when she sought care.

After we had our first child, the migraines continued to worsen. At this point, nothing seemed to help, and she was in near-constant misery. We saw several specialists, including neurologists, hormone specialists, and pain specialists, but no one seemed to have a truly effective plan.

Desperate, I contacted researchers around the country who studied migraines and asked for their help. An angel of a doctor from Texas named Dr. Stuart Black responded. We had our first conversation with Dr. Black, chief of neurology at Baylor University Medical Center at Dallas, in a hospital hallway while Brianna was hospitalized for another migraine exacerbation. He advised us to see Dr. Mark Green at Mount Sinai in the Upper East Side of Manhattan.

Dr. Green was our first step in her healing from migraines. He was a master clinician, a true healer in the area of migraines and headaches. He was also a genuinely kind-hearted man. He explained that with migraines, the last one in some ways causes the next one because the headache pain induces changes in the brain that make it even more susceptible to migraines in the future. He made recommendations that were not in any of the textbooks or scientific articles I'd read, but they gradually helped put more and more space between Brianna and her migraines . . . first a sliver, then a little more.

With space, we were able to try other treatments, and those other treatments were more likely to work now than in the past because she wasn't constantly under bombardment from recurrent migraines. She was gradually improving, and the interval between emergency department visits got longer and longer.

One day, she was well enough to come with me to an American Heart Association conference in Orlando, Florida, where I was presenting some of my research with a mentor, Dr. Pamela Douglas of Duke University. This trip changed our lives. As soon as we arrived, it was as if Brianna were a different person: no debilitating migraines, no severe pain, and tremendously more energy. We took our only child at the time and spent a day at Disney. She was able to push the stroller around and have a full day of activity—something I had not seen since she first became pregnant. We were both surprised and heartened.

When we returned to New York, she had a debilitating migraine the very next day. I couldn't believe it, and I vowed in that very moment to leave the Northeast. I began looking for a new job in Florida or a region with stable weather, since weather changes—and thunderstorms in particular—were at least one controllable migraine trigger for Brianna.

I interviewed at universities in Florida and California and received job offers, but ultimately, I decided to join the faculty of UCLA. By the time we moved, Brianna was pregnant with our second boy.

At UCLA, my career accelerated. I won the first of four large NIH grants that would eventually pave the path to my tenure. My research focused on clinical trials and behavioral economic interventions for cardiovascular disease prevention.

The first study tested a weight-loss intervention for low-income, obese adults; the second tested an intervention to reduce cardiovascular risk among people with HIV; the third tested a smoking cessation intervention in safety-net hospital systems; and the fourth was a large study launched in conjunction with the LA County health system to reduce rates of uncontrolled hypertension among low-income Angelenos. Through these projects, I deepened my expertise in working with health systems and private organizations in the pursuit of public health goals.

My work was going well, and Brianna's health was steadily improving. Day by day, she saw incremental improvements in the frequency and severity of her migraines. Days spent completely incapacitated and recovering from a migraine at home were becoming less and less common. When our second boy was born, she was able to do more as a mom than she could with our first little guy.

Meanwhile, less illness from severe migraines and less time recovering in bed also meant she had fewer buffers from the parts of me that felt unsafe and afraid. I was still working with a therapist, but the changes were too small and minute to keep pace with the stress my problems were creating for our relationship, and for my relationship with our kids.

I explored some of what we went through, and how people can learn from our experience, in an article for the *Washington Post* in 2016:

> *As a doctor, I thought I knew how to treat my patients. Then my wife ended up in the hospital. Here's what her illness taught me about successful medical care.*

I've spent all my professional life as a doctor. But when my wife suffered a chronic, debilitating illness, I realized that medicine looks totally different through the eyes of a patient. Our experience—through seven hospitalizations, countless more emergency department visits and endless doctors' appointments—taught me lessons about surviving the American health-care system that I could never have learned in a classroom or in my professional role. The things I learned continue to shape how I now care for my patients.

Here are the points that stick with me still:

1. **Speak up.** During one hospitalization, my wife complained of pain in her arm at the site of an intravenous catheter that had been placed for hydration. The nurse reassured us that all was fine, but her pain persisted and gradually worsened. We could have insisted that the IV be re-checked or removed, but not wanting to be perceived as "too demanding," I decided to back down. The next day, she developed thrombophlebitis—painful inflammation of blood vessels—at the IV site. She was too sick to advocate for herself at the time. My choice to acquiesce contributed to her avoidable suffering.

These types of situations happen often in my experience: the man who is hospitalized with a heart attack but wants to discuss his foot pain, or the woman treated for pneumonia whose primary concern is her anxiety. Earlier in my career, I paid less attention to these issues when they didn't seem related to my patients' major medical problems, but I rarely make that mistake now. Even if I don't immediately have an answer to my patient's problem, I try and file the issue away and revisit it the next time I see the patient. As the physician and scholar Sir William Osler famously said, "Listen to your patient, he is telling you the diagnosis."

2. Don't be afraid to ask for a specialist. My wife was, at times, in excruciating pain. In fact, memories of her lying in misery while her doctors tried in vain to relieve her suffering are some of the saddest of my life. It was only the unconventional treatment choices of two specialists in distinct disciplines—one a neurologist, the other a pain specialist—that helped loosen the suffocating grip of her pain.

This experience reiterated how important it is to bring in specialists. And it reminded me how valuable pain management is. As an internist, most of my training in pain management happened on the job while caring for patients with cancer. Though I picked up strategies from more experienced nurse practitioners and physicians, I don't have nearly the expertise of specialists, who receive formal training in a range of interventions and therapies. They also spend more time with patients suffering from chronic, painful conditions and learn through these interactions how to better aid their suffering.

The perspective of pain-management specialists is particularly important, because many physicians don't treat pain seriously enough. In my experience, private conversations among doctors about patients with pain are often dominated by terms like "drug-seeking" and "addicts." The stigma surrounding pain treatment is so powerful that doctors frequently bring these biases with them into meetings with patients, quickly turning a conversation's tone from friendly to adversarial. This can leave patients feeling neglected, ignored or ashamed. Now, when I take care of patients for whom pain is a major component of their medical presentation, I am more diligent about explicitly addressing whether my pain management plan is likely to be effective. If I have doubts, I almost invariably consult a pain specialist.

3. Don't feel bad about asking to speak with a patient advocate. Patient advocates—sometimes called patient representatives—listen and respond to patients' concerns about their care and often address concerns about quality or communication breakdowns. Discussing your concerns with them tends to focus the attention of doctors and hospital leaders in a way that might otherwise not be possible.

We used a patient advocate once during my wife's care. A change in hospital leadership created an administrative roadblock that prevented one of her primary doctors from caring for her. We felt that the urgency of her needs were being cast aside, and I contacted a patient advocate and wrote a letter to the hospital's president and executives. The issue was subsequently resolved.

I've also seen patient advocates work as a doctor. Recently, the family of a critically ill patient I cared for contacted a patient advocate because they were upset that more aggressive treatments had not been initiated by one of the specialists involved in her care—a concern I had picked up on in my conversations with them but had not fully appreciated. Managing her treatment alongside the specialists who were also involved was my top priority, but the advocate sharpened my attention, and I became more engaged in the specialist's decision-making. Ultimately, she did receive more aggressive therapy, which speeded her recovery.

4. Share your health challenges with others and don't stop searching for help. Of the many lessons I learned while my wife was sick, this might be the most important one. I searched endlessly for help from my physician colleagues, books, medical journals and websites, seeking ways to relieve my loved one's suffering. Though many of these efforts led to dead ends, salvation finally came in the form of a senior neurologist in Texas who was kind enough to respond to an email I sent him. He had suggestions about how to manage her care and ideas about treatments to try, most of which we pursued. Additionally, he connected us to a preeminent neurologist in New York whose new, unconventional ideas finally began helping her and gave her relief.

As a doctor, it was undoubtedly easier for me to reach out to physician colleagues and make sense of the scientific literature than it will probably be for those not in the medical field. I encourage those without a medical background to speak with acquaintances who are doctors or nurses, or nonmedical friends who have experienced the health-care system firsthand as either a caregiver or patient. The Hippocratic Oath obliges us to help when we can, and you never know who may have had a similar experience or what another physician might be willing to do to help you.

CHAPTER 4

Getting Free

Professionally, I was excelling, but personally, I was struggling. Despite seeking help from a therapist and making incremental improvements, I remained a fearful being at my core.

Emails from my supervisor would rattle me before I even read their contents. Social situations would leave me fearful about saying or doing the "wrong" thing and experiencing shame and embarrassment. Every new idea Brianna proposed, from things as simple as going to a concert or as complex as planning a vacation, would leave me frightful about finances. If I was the only black student in one of my graduate school classes, I would hesitate to raise my hand, fearful that I might leave a negative impression by asking a question that was perceived as unintelligent.

Fear was my front-seat passenger, but I hid it well from public view with a commanding control over my facial expressions and body language. However, there was no hiding from Brianna. Her fine-tuned senses and intuition perceived every dark impulse and fear-based survival strategy I employed. The experience gradually wore her down over the years, as she dealt with my frequent "freak-outs," a term she sometimes used to describe them. Eventually, she told me she felt like I was "putting her light out." It was heartbreaking for me to hear.

Ironically, despite my emotional struggles, I never felt as much courage and peace as I did when I was with her. Looking back, I know this was because love rouses the most graceful parts of our being. I had both light and dark stirring within me, and while the former was ultimately more powerful, the latter was dominating the relationship between Brianna and me.

Brianna always traveled in a more spiritual plane, and her world was characterized by intuitive insights, deep connections with a few soul sisters that transcended my understanding of what relationships were, and a history of extraordinary experiences that were hard to explain with natural laws. This created contrast between us: I was fearful, while she was naturally fearless. My work and profession lay firmly in the physical and scientific domains, while she primarily devoted her attention to the emotional and spiritual domains. I was emotionally fragile, while she was incredibly emotionally resilient.

Nonetheless, the burden of dealing with my emotional fragility without a respite for years was too much. By 2019, Brianna was terribly worn down, and our relationship was at its lowest point. I had worked hard, sought help, and put a tremendous amount of energy into pursuing emotional healthiness, but it was not even close to enough. Inside, I felt a growing sense of hopelessness and helplessness; as much as I loved Brianna, what difference did it make if I was making her miserable?

Then one day, Brianna came home and said something she'd never said before. "I found someone I want you to see. He helps people with the type of trauma you went through as a child. I think he can help you."

Like many people who need help with a personal issue, my initial reaction was resistance. I wanted to get better, but part of me was lazy. My resistance only grew when I learned how much it would cost to work with him.

But Brianna was certain I needed to see him. And considering what I had put her through over the years, I knew I had no choice but to agree. Before I met him, I read a book he had written, *Free for Life*. While I could not comprehend all of its contents, I began sensing that he knew exactly what he was talking about.

We scheduled a phone call, and I emptied my wheelbarrow of skepticism at his doorstep, which seemed only to amuse him. Shortly thereafter, in the second week of December 2019, I went to see him in Marina Del Rey for the five-day program he offered to beginners. The program was comprised of two sessions a day, each lasting about two hours. His name is Christopher Maher.

Christopher is a former Navy SEAL who experienced profound trauma as a child. As a young adult, he pushed his life and his body to destructive limits and from this place of pain ultimately discovered a path toward true healing. To help people remove their stress, tension, and trauma, he uses a combination of ancient techniques that were developed by others and new techniques that he developed himself.

The broad range of techniques that he uses when working with people include *Ma Xing*; *Body of Light*; destressing and detensing body work that involves isometric, concentric, and eccentric contractions; and destressing and detensing exercises that an individual can engage in daily after their week with him ends.

Much of his work is based in Chinese meridian theory, and the qualities of *chi* and energy. Related to this, one of the lines from his book that, to me, captured how he helps people was based on an age-old saying from Chinese medicine: "Where there is pain, there is no flow; where there is no flow, pain is sure to follow." My sense is that this adage is not solely about physical pain, but also about emotional and spiritual pain.

On the first day, we started by discussing what I wanted to get out of the week. We also did some body work and then used a tool he developed called *Body of Light* to begin addressing my childhood sexual trauma. Christopher described this as a "verbal-based energetic system used to help people reintegrate and locate the energies, consciousness, and projections that keep their bodies, brains, and nervous systems out of alignment." I was skeptical and told Christopher as much, and when I left his apartment that day, I felt that nothing had really changed. In fact, the only distinct feeling I remember having was annoyance that I had probably wasted my money.

I went to bed that evening and awoke hours later, in the middle of the night. I still remember that moment well. When I awoke, I could feel that something was different . . . a strange sensation that I couldn't quite put my finger on. It was as if something had been lifted out of my chest, leaving a lightness in its place, a felicity, an ease. It was curious, but I didn't know what to make of it. I went back to sleep and awoke the next morning.

That morning, it became very clear to me that something was indeed different. With three little boys—who were one, three, and six years old at that time—to care for, school drop-off, work responsibilities, and everything else in our lives, I was always a nervous wreck in the morning, rushing to get everyone clean, fed, and out the door on time with my wife. That morning, the nervousness was gone. I was actually enjoying my kids, and we were having—for the first time on a school day ever—a jolly morning together. After breakfast, I remember pulling Brianna aside and excitedly saying, "Honey, every day I'm always freaking out when it's time to leave to take the boys to school. I'm always worried we will not have enough time. But I'm not freaking out right now!" She smiled.

After dropping the boys off at school, I took an Uber to Christopher's place. I started chatting with the driver and proceeded to have the very first conversation in my adult life in which I genuinely connected emotionally with a stranger. I was STUNNED. We talked about his family and his life, and I couldn't believe how present I felt, and how real and in the moment I felt. I genuinely and authentically cared about him, about his well-being, and about his relationship with his loved ones. I had never experienced anything like this in my life.

As I write this, I stare at the words with some incredulity. What had I been doing in my interactions with other people for all those years before? The truth is I was doing the best I could with the facilities I had. But trauma cuts us off from our being, our true selves, and makes something that should be the most natural thing in the world—emotion connection with other human beings—impossible to access. Babies come out of the womb understanding almost nothing about the world other than how to connect with others through the language of love, yet with all of my education and career success, I had never been able to do this.

Every individual's reaction to stress and trauma is unique, but when it is lifted away, what remains for each of us is ease and grace where the injury once lived.

When I arrived at Christopher's apartment, I thanked him profusely. "If we stopped now and did not do one more thing, it would be worth it," I told him, jokingly referring to my complaints about the price of the week's sessions. He smiled and laughed because, as I would later learn, he had helped thousands of people burdened by stress, tension, and trauma, and he knew exactly what was going to happen to me when I left his apartment the day before.

Thankfully, though, we did not stop there. As miraculous as it sounds, things just got better and better. On the second day, we started a technique called *Ma Xing*. During this technique, Christopher walked up and down the backs of my thighs as I lay down. The discomfort I experienced as he stomped on me was intense, and I went from feeling acute pain to feeling a sense of enjoyment, and—as incredible as it must sound—at one point, I even felt like a tiger.

Christopher explained that this was my spirit animal. As I learned from him, *Ma Xing* engages the urinary bladder channel, which is the master channel in Chinese meridian theory. Further, he explained that this channel has access to every aspect of a human being's behavior and thoughts, including their mind, brain, physical being, spiritual energy, and emotional intelligence.

We continued with a combination of *Mao Xing*; body work that involved isometric, concentric, and eccentric contractions; and *Body of Light* exercises to strip away layers of stress and tension that I had built up over the years. As they fell away, so did the fears I had developed in response to stress and trauma.

By the end of the week, I was literally a new man. I felt euphoria, as if I had been granted a new state of being. Even now, it remains an experience that is the closest thing to a "miracle" I have ever experienced in my life. And to this day, I don't truly understand why these methods were effective for me, but I have always been a guy who was more interested in results than in fully grasping how they came to be.

Christopher helped me understand that the euphoria would continue as the lifetime of fear that lay deep within me was transmuted into love. Later, even as I transitioned into less euphoric states, the feeling of freedom continued.

It was an unbelievable experience.

Christopher remained a guide, teaching me new destressing and detensing exercises I could practice at home to continue my transformation, providing feedback on the number of repetitions of these exercises to do as my life evolved, and providing other insights and guidance. I was incredibly grateful, yet simultaneously incredulous about the experience—and my new experience of life. I am immeasurably grateful to Brianna for finding him for us and will remain so for all the days I walk this Earth.

And while she was overjoyed that we had finally found a solution, she was also exhausted, like a warrior who had been running on adrenalin and finally stopped moving. All that she had done to emotionally support me and our kids over the years and keep them healthy, despite my toxicity, had caught up with her. Fortunately, she worked with Christopher two months later and emerged stronger, more insightful, and more powerful than ever.

Though we did not realize it at the time, we would soon discover that the timing of our work with Christopher was divine and guided by the hand of providence. Early in 2020, news about a novel coronavirus was penetrating health media, and a cloud of fear was slowly settling over the country.

CHAPTER 5

Caught Unprepared

COVID-19 presented an extraordinary challenge for public health decision making. There was tremendous uncertainty about which parts of our country would be affected, how severely, whether the scenes of hospital overload that were first seen in Wuhan, China, and then in Italy might unfold here, and which policy measures would be effective.

My initial reaction was skepticism about the pandemic's potential impact. This skepticism was borne out of experience. At this point in my medical career, I had already seen a handful of pandemic false alarms come and go, and I am a somewhat skeptical guy by nature.

But as I studied reports on the morbidity and mortality countries were facing, watched scientific presentations about the experience from the front lines (Massachusetts General Hospital, for example, presented a very enlightening grand rounds presentation from doctors in Wuhan), and pored over news articles, I grew to feel that we were, in fact, preparing to enter an extraordinary period. This was crystallized when startling and tragic reports of completely besieged and overwhelmed hospitals in New York City appeared on the evening news.

Still, I was averse to the cloud of fear and anxiety that was settling into the country and, in fact, the world. Brianna and I felt similarly, although my own experience would doubtlessly have been different had I not worked with Christopher. I truly don't know how I would have felt. I likely would have been too out of touch with my emotions to take in the full emotional effect of what was happening, but simultaneously not healthy enough to clearly recognize that fear was an emotion to be rejected because it was anathema to life, love, and freedom. But fortunately, I will never know.

As a clinical researcher at UCLA, I spent about 20 percent of my time caring for patients at Ronald Reagan UCLA Medical Center in the beautiful Westwood neighborhood of West Los Angeles. This hospital was one of the best at which I had ever worked, offering highly technical care to complex patients, including many organ transplant patients. I happened to be scheduled to work in the middle of March 2019.

During that week, I witnessed a panicked hospital for the first time in my life. Protocols that were intended to protect medical staff members, such as mask and face shield protocols, changed almost daily, and communications from leadership at the hospital were punctuated with an unspoken franticness. My team, which included medical residents, took care of some of the hospital's first patients with COVID-19. My residents were terrified.

One young woman had been diagnosed with COVID-19, but her most serious ailment was anxiety, directly related to watching news about the virus on TV, as she would later tell me. She had been admitted because of an abnormal chest x-ray, but her findings were not consistent with pneumonia. The nursing staff urged me to discharge her as soon as possible, and I agreed. The major medical therapy I provided to her was counseling and reassurance.

A second, an older man, had been diagnosed with COVID-19 while undergoing chemotherapy. He was also not seriously ill. The hospital enrolled him in one of the inpatient treatment protocols, and he remained stable during his hospitalization. He was fairly stoic, but that did not surprise me. Patients who battle cancer often have tremendous grit, and I had seen that demonstrated time and time again during my career. Other patients we saw that week with suspected or confirmed COVID-19 were more seriously ill, and most of these patients were being cared for in the intensive care unit.

Personally, I was worried about taking on the health risks associated with caring for patients with a novel disease. I was worried that I could become ill, but I accepted long ago that that was part of my career choice. However, as a clinical researcher, I wanted to know what the data showed. Fortunately, case fatality data from Wuhan were already widely available.

One afternoon after rounds, I sat down with my team to review some of these data. It was clear from case fatality rates in Wuhan that this was a disease whose morbidity was concentrated in older people. The case fatality rate among children in Wuhan was basically zero, and the case fatality rate among young people—like the 20-something-year-old medical students and residents on my team—was also close to zero. I found the data reassuring. The residents on my team were not persuaded. I remember thinking, "Wow, fear is powerful."

That month also saw the beginning of lockdowns in California, as Governor Newsom announced on March 19, 2019, that the state would be shutting down. The debate among parents about whether to keep our kids' schools open was suddenly highjacked by the announcement, and Brianna and I began scrambling to figure out childcare.

After work in the evenings, I would talk to her about the environment in the hospital, the heavy climate of fear and panic, and the fear that was also permeating my residents and society. We both saw it for the evil and destructiveness it represented. Brianna's clarity about the pandemic was an incredibly valuable North Star for me, as the panic of the hospital would sometimes leave me with doubts about the wisdom of our perspective. She never had doubts.

Yearning to contribute a reasonable perspective to a difficult situation, I drafted an op-ed for submission to a newspaper. Brianna edited it, and it was published in *USA Today* a few days later.

The message was simple: in all likelihood, harm was coming—this was unavoidable. Risk was most acute among the oldest members of our society, but there was little that could be effectively done to prevent them from contracting a contagious respiratory virus, as world history had repeatedly demonstrated and clinical epidemiology strongly suggested. Finally, the costs of mitigation efforts—particularly school and business closures—could eventually be enormous, so the lockdowns that were being proposed were a very dangerous policy option. Therefore, the wisest strategy was to build up hospital treatment capacity and pivot back to sustaining and supporting society and living.

This first article garnered significant attention, and I felt satisfaction from the sense of exerting a positive impact on an important policy issue that many leading thinkers in medicine and public health were getting wrong. As unrealistic pronouncements suggesting that the virus could be contained continued to fill op-ed pages in the *New York Times* and the *Washington Post*, it seemed time to write a second article.

After Brianna edited it, I submitted the article to the *Wall Street Journal,* and they published it immediately. In "Lockdowns Won't Stop the Spread," the message was captured by the title. I laid out the scientific and social reasons lockdowns were bound to fail, and why accepting this reality would help us move toward a more sustainable, sensible, and humane approach to navigating the pandemic.

This article received even more attention than its predecessor, and I heard from colleagues around the nation who expressed gratitude for its message. Many felt similarly but were afraid to be vocal due to concerns about reprisals. By this time, the politicization of the pandemic and the hardening of prolockdown positions were just setting in.

While I thought the practicality of suggesting that we abandon tactics that were not only untenable, but would cause needless suffering, and focus on saving the most lives while keeping society intact would be a welcome perspective amidst the growing madness, I could never have predicted what followed.

Coronavirus Pandemic: We Were Caught Unprepared. It Is Too Late for Shutdowns to Save Us.[*]
USA Today, March 24, 2020

What we should do is to keep shutdowns short, keep the economy going and build our public health system for the pandemic.

---

[*] https://www.usatoday.com/story/opinion/2020/03/24/coronavirus-shutdowns-worth-public-health-system-unprepared
-column/2898324001/.

"When we see ourselves in a situation which must be endured and gone through, it is best to make up our minds to it. Meet it with firmness, and accommodate everything to it in the best way practicable. This lessens the evil, while fretting and fuming only serves to increase your own torment." —Thomas Jefferson

We are fretting and we are fuming. As a country, we have been caught miserably flat-footed after receiving warnings about what lay ahead when cases of Covid-19 began exploding in Wuhan, China. Messages from local and state leaders about how to respond to the pandemic change almost daily—a sure sign they have no idea what they are doing. Shutdowns are happening here in California and in New York, and will probably spread to the rest of the nation.

I spent the past week taking care of patients with Covid-19 at UCLA's flagship hospital, and the atmosphere there is, appropriately, one of crisis—like other hospitals around the country. Before we bend to the next reactionary spasms of our political leaders, let's take a look at what we know.

Epidemiologists around the world have studied patterns of our social contacts, studied our population density and studied the Covid-19 virus' transmission characteristics. For better or worse, we actually have a lot of data to work with, thanks to the countries that have already been struck hard. Additionally, epidemiologists have been accurately modeling disease outbreaks for years. As someone who spent extra time in medical school to earn a Ph.D. focused on economics, statistics and decision analysis, I feel confident about the epidemiologists' projections.

Shutdowns can't save overwhelmed hospitals

Here's the problem: Because of the (understandable) fear and hysteria of the moment, few U.S. leaders are seriously talking about the endgame. The epidemiologic models I've seen indicate that the shutdowns and school closures will temporarily slow the virus' spread, but when they're lifted, we will essentially emerge right back where we started. And, by the way, no matter what, our hospitals will still be overwhelmed. There has already been too much community spread to prevent this inevitability.

We don't have a totalitarian government like China, and we value our civil liberties too much to take the measures (i.e., total lockdown) that would be needed to rapidly decrease the infection rate to zero. This means that, even with shutdowns, the virus will still spread. Unfortunately, this also means that rates of "community immunity," often referred to as "herd immunity," will slow. As a result, we will always be vulnerable to the virus spreading rapidly again as soon as shutdown measures are lifted, unless they are immediately reimplemented—over and over and over again.

The only potential savior that would prevent this scenario is an effective vaccine, but the estimates I've seen put us 12–18 months away from making that a reality. Clinical trials are underway and will hopefully yield effective treatment, but a cure is unlikely. Either way, the models indicate that our hospitals, at current capacity, will be overwhelmed, with or without shutdowns.

As Americans, we could, if we set our minds to it, stay locked down for 18 months—but we won't. Can you imagine a United States in which children are forced to forgo proper schooling, unemployment and poverty decimate millions more lives, and our economy is strangled into a persistent depression? And all for a virus that, when all is said and done, most people will recover from— even the elderly (death rates are highest in adults older than 80, at 10-20%)? The lockdown cost will be staggering—far more costly than Covid-19's horrific wrath. This terrible trade-off is the path upon which we've set ourselves because our public health system was unprepared for a pandemic.

Please don't believe politicians who say we can control this pandemic with a few weeks of shutdown. None of the models I've seen (or history's teachings, or common sense) supports this as a possibility. As soon as restrictions are lifted, the virus will once again tear through our communities with abandon, until one day (hopefully) we have an effective vaccine. To contain a virus with shutdowns, you must either go big—which is what China did—or you don't go at all. In this country, we hold liberty too dearly to go big; eventually, citizens will push back—hard.

Focus on economy and health care system

Tragically, over the coming weeks, as the numbers of people sickened and killed by Covid-19 increase—and they will—the resulting fear and the hysteria will be used to try to prolong the shutdowns. This move might work in some states that lean left, but states that lean right will resist. Short of a miracle, expect to see a tragedy unlike anything we've seen in generations. Heartbreakingly, people you know will die. Celebrities and politicians we all know will die. Hospitals will be overwhelmed and helpless.

Here is my prescription for local and state leaders: Keep shutdowns short, keep the economy going, keep schools in session, keep jobs intact, and focus single-mindedly on building the capacity we need to survive this into our health care system.

We desperately need more intensive care unit beds and ventilators to give the severely ill a chance of survival: Borrow them, buy them, build them, convert structures to coronavirus-dedicated centers, etc. We must do whatever is necessary—and do it yesterday. And for heaven's sake, where on earth are the Covid-19 tests?

At this point, no matter what we do, we tragically will lose many Americans. Short of a miracle treatment, it's too late for any other outcome. However, our economy, people's jobs and livelihoods, and the education of our children should not become collateral damage. We must not let ill-informed, fear-fueled policy compound the casualties of Covid-19.

Lockdowns Won't Stop the Spread*
Wall Street Journal, April 9, 2020

Stopping the coronavirus and protecting the economy are one and the same, but it is too late to do either.

The pandemic crisis now rests on a fulcrum. On one side is Covid-19 and every possible action that might prevent people from contracting and dying from infection. On the other side is everything else that matters: livelihoods that allow people to feed and shelter their families; civil liberties; the education of children; social well-being, including the prevention of loneliness, isolation and domestic violence; and all other medical conditions, from cancer and heart disease to dental emergencies. The belief that it is worth sacrificing anything and everything at the altar of flattening the coronavirus curve is foolish. But many leaders are behaving that way. We need a clearer picture of all that is at stake before those at the helm burn down the village to save it.

Examples of bad actions, often by well-intentioned leaders, are proliferating. The mayor of Chicago warned joggers that a stay-at-home order means they may not go on long runs without risking arrest, a flagrant disregard for the American values of liberty and prudence, not to mention the common-sense benefits of exercise. A city in Texas threatens to fine residents up to $1,000 if they (and their children) don't wear masks in public. New Jersey Gov. Phil Murphy recommends a policy of social distancing within your own household. "Keep your distance between yourself and other family members," he cautioned recently. More broadly, governors have ordered shutdowns to slow the coronavirus without acknowledging what these shutdowns cost.

Encouragingly, this has also been a time of extraordinary action by private citizens. The largest volunteer network in New York, New

---

* https://www.wsj.com/articles/lockdowns-wont-stop-the-spread-11586474560.

York Cares, decided that instead of closing up shop, it will press on to serve the community. Grocery stores have created special shopping hours for seniors and health-care workers. The New England Patriots used its team plane to fly a million N95 masks from China to Boston. The list of courageous acts is lengthy.

To help set the right course for our country, we must grasp some simple—but tough—facts. The novel coronavirus is highly contagious and tragically lethal to many. There is no guarantee of a vaccine within the next 18 months. We have taken measures to slow the virus, but these can't stop it. The only thing that can stop the virus at this advanced stage of community transmission is a complete lockdown, which can happen in authoritarian countries like China, but not in the U.S.

Are shutdowns enough? No. Despite the efforts, there is still enough human contact to ensure the virus will spread. Take a look at the long list of "essential" services and exemptions on California's Covid-19 website, for example. Shutdowns will cause the virus to spread more slowly, but it will spread nonetheless.

When shutdowns end, the virus will spread and Covid-19 deaths will increase. Without a vaccine and community immunity—often called "herd immunity"—this outcome is all but guaranteed. The only thing that will temporarily quell it in the near term, short of a miracle treatment, is another shutdown. But states will get only one pass at this. Once lifted, the appetite for a repeat shutdown will be tepid at best, even in left-leaning states. The reality of the shutdown's costs—the upheaval caused by school closures, economic hurt, social isolation and lost lives and livelihoods—will be fresh. Some argue that stopping Covid-19 and protecting the economy are one and the same. Although this is true, it is too late to do either.

Accepting this reality will help us make better decisions. The modeling predicts that the number of sick patients is likely to be profound and exceed anything seen in generations. It's therefore clear that building health-care capacity—adding hospital beds, converting and building coronavirus-only treatment facilities and sourcing ventilators—is the right step to take.

Embracing reality also makes other things clear. If we can't shut down for 18 months on the gamble that an effective vaccine will arrive, how long will it be worth committing millions of families to poverty and uprooting lives, education and every other part of the economy? Politicians have largely dodged this question.

Already, ethicists are helping us think about how to allocate ventilators when hospitals run short. And how many older doctors and nurses have to die before we seriously discuss allowing older health-care workers—say, above 59—to opt out of dangerous settings like emergency departments and hospital wards? My experience caring for patients with suspected or diagnosed Covid-19 infections at UCLA has made it clear to me that treating them in the same setting as patients with other diagnoses is unsafe, even with personal protective equipment.

Many difficult decisions lie ahead. We stand the best chance of making good decisions if we consider everything at stake, and not only the singular goal of reducing Covid-19 deaths.

CHAPTER 6

Seeing Through the Lockdowns

We all remember pivotal moments when we learn something is not what we think it is, or bear witness to a revelation that forever changes how we see something. And once something is seen, it cannot be unseen. The incident that forever changed my view of the pandemic occurred in late April 2020.

A few days earlier, I had stumbled across a video of a recent Tucker Carlson monologue from his *Tucker Carlson Tonight* show in which he was discussing the pandemic. I came across it quite by chance, as we did not have cable and, prior to the pandemic, my exposure to Tucker was limited to when he would stir up enough controversy to be covered by mainstream media and news channels. Now, I am a big fan of Tucker and watch YouTube clips of his show frequently. But back then, I felt differently.

With some shame, I have to confess that the mainstream media's campaign against him had had some traction with me. I wish I had been more conscious of their strategies, which were ultimately attempts to subvert his voice by creating sufficient amounts of public outrage to cost him advertisers and—they hoped—his show. And while I tended to be fairly resistant to harboring feelings of "outrage," their campaigns against him had succeeded in casting him in a slightly negative light in my mind.

But this video somehow came across my computer, and I listened to Tucker talk about how the lockdowns were really an exercise in political power. As he spoke, it was as if something my subconscious self knew suddenly snapped right into my consciousness. *He is exactly right*, I remember thinking. The fact that a desire for political domination was a major motivation for early pandemic decisions is widely recognized now, but Tucker was prescient in his observation that day, as he continues to be on other issues in the present. And his words forever changed my perspective on pandemic politics.

Days later, as I settled at my desk to work that evening after putting the kids to bed with Brianna, I came across a news article. There was a story about a woman in San Diego who had organized a protest to oppose stay-at-home orders.

As if nothing unusual were happening, the reporter described how the San Diego Police Department was planning to charge her for protesting. My jaw dropped. A woman in the United States was peacefully protesting for nothing more than her freedom, and the power of the state was being mobilized to strip her of this right, to intimidate her and others like her. My soul felt crushed by the injustice.

I am fortunate to have always had an innate appreciation for freedom, and ever since working with Christopher and removing the emotional and spiritual clutter that filled my life and clouded my judgment, that appreciation had grown clearer and stronger than ever. Freedom is our connection to God and the lifeblood of our souls. I was aghast that police officers saw nothing wrong with taking that right away from this woman for simply expressing herself peacefully. Not only is this a right protected by the U.S. Constitution, it is a natural right afforded by divinity to every human being through the fact that we are reflections of God.

My indignation transformed to tears as I sat that evening in front of my computer and reflected on the woman's circumstances and where we were as a country and a people. I knew what I had to write about next.

That moment, I drafted an article that discussed how it was not only immoral and unjust, but also unwise, to cast aside civil liberties during a pandemic, because doing so would incite tremendous resistance. This would clearly be the case because, for many people, their souls interpret infringements on civil liberties as a life-or-death struggle. I submitted it to the *Wall Street Journal*, which printed it a few days later.

Like the prior article I published, this article received a substantial amount of attention, and individuals from within and outside the medical community contacted me. Almost uniformly, these individuals expressed appreciation for my recognition of the harms to civil liberties that were unfolding. One of my colleagues at UCLA expressed bewilderment at the fact that I anticipated this development. "How did you know?" she asked.

In polite words that I can't quite recall, I basically responded by saying that it was obvious. In retrospect, though, what her comments belied was how disconnected many members of the medical community were from civil liberties and natural rights. That disconnection—later plainly demonstrated by how eagerly doctors latched on to broad mandates for new, unapproved vaccines—was a critical contributing factor in the many public health leadership failures during the pandemic.

Around this time, Brianna and I began a lockdown tradition that we continued until a few weeks prior to our departure from Los Angeles in September 2021. As any parent of young children knows, as much as you love the little guys, they can be all-consuming of your time, energy, and attention, leaving little at the end of the day for emotional intimacy and connection with your spouse. Lockdowns that close schools only make things worse.

So often, the only way to preserve that intimacy and connection is to deliberately carve out time to create it. With that in mind, Brianna and I started having Tuesday brunch dates while our energetic and physically active boys were at the park with their babysitters. We visited different parts of Los Angeles every week, going to downtown LA, Beverly Hills, West Hollywood, Santa Monica, you name it. We would select the part of town we wanted to visit and pick a cuisine, and let fate handle the rest.

At first, because of the Los Angeles lockdown, all we could order was takeout. So, we would take our food to a park or the beach, and sometimes we would just park and eat in the car. Our conversations were dominated by whatever was happening with the pandemic, and we would discuss new policies that were being enacted, how unwise or misinformed (or both) leaders were, and what forces and motivations were truly driving decision making. These dates with Brianna are some of my favorite memories from the pandemic. We truly had such an enjoyable time during our miniescapes. The conversations we had on our dates also happened to be the creative force behind nearly every article I published during the pandemic.

During one of our Tuesday dates in May, we talked about the growing clamor for reopening. While we were obviously supportive of everyone getting back to life, we knew reopening would be problematic, because so many businesses and political leaders were still holding on to the illusion that safety protocols for businesses would somehow succeed in "containing" the virus.

The foolishness of this position was further underscored by the fact that case counts were actually trending up already in Los Angeles—while we were still deep in lockdown. At this point in the pandemic, I thought (hoped) that policymakers might listen to reason. With this in mind, I wrote an article explaining that reopening efforts would only be sustainable if businesses prepared themselves for the inevitable—that the virus would continue spreading, just as it had during the lockdowns, and some people would become sick.

The lesson that the article aimed to convey was that, despite the tragedy of illness, what we were losing in life—disrupting kids' schooling and education, forcing young people to put their dreams on hold, and pushing small businesses and the families that owned them to the brink of extinction—was not worth what we might be saving in deaths. Brianna edited it, and it appeared in the *Wall Street Journal* on May 21, 2020.

I was admittedly disappointed when it seemed like my words fell on deaf ears. Almost no one seemed to care, and yet, reopenings were bound to fail if this issue was not addressed. At least part of the reason that the public health community proved incapable of communicating realistic expectations to the public was the disorienting effect of fear on the consciousness of so many of their leaders. Brianna and I felt that professionals in public health were basically engaged in an elaborate game of wishful thinking.

California began reopening in late May and early June. A few weeks later, unfortunately—but not surprisingly—businesses started closing just as quickly as they reopened. Predictably, the closures were implemented in response to the governor's claims of rising COVID case counts and hospitalizations. It was frustrating to watch, and it set the backdrop for the hyperpoliticization that was just around the corner.

The Looming Civil-Liberties Battle*
Wall Street Journal, April 29, 2020

The stage is set for a post-shutdown showdown between personal freedom and public health.

The battle against Covid-19 is gradually morphing into a battle over civil liberties. Just as the first phase of the coronavirus struggle has been consequential for lives and livelihoods, the next phase of lifting shutdowns will have similar gravity.

According to a recent Associated Press-NORC Center for Public Affairs Research poll, most of the American public supports stay-at-home orders, and more people think there should be greater rather than lighter restrictions. But a substantial minority of Americans are concerned about the legitimacy of shutdown orders and the sensibility of extending them, with protests stretching from North Carolina to California. These protesters have largely been dismissed—or, worse, arrested and pursued for criminal prosecution. This will intensify concerns about heavy-handedness, energize the efforts of dissenters, and jeopardize the effectiveness of future public-health efforts.

The civil liberties issues raised by the Covid-19 pandemic range from the basic, such as whether government can stop you from

---

* https://www.wsj.com/articles/the-looming-civil-liberties-battle-11588198523.

leaving your house or opening your business, to the ludicrous, such as whether Michigan Gov. Gretchen Whitmer can say it's OK for you to launch your rowboat but not your motorboat (an order she has since reversed). When a surfer in the ocean is arrested for violating stay-at-home orders in Southern California, or a father in Colorado is arrested for not social distancing while playing with his wife and child at a park, or two women in San Diego County are targeted for prosecution after organizing shutdown protests, it's clear that something other than public health is at play.

The only reason these incidents didn't receive sunlight commensurate with their indecency is that Covid-19-induced terror has hijacked the nation. This is a country whose deepest roots lie in the soil of liberty and freedom, values that have catalyzed the most important social and cultural movements in modern history. Epidemiologic studies of the population prevalence of novel coronavirus antibodies are pointing to much higher rates of infection than previously thought—with the corollary that mortality is much lower. Surely, as fear loosens its grip—and there is evidence from that same AP-NORC poll that this is happening—these overreaches, and those still to come, will reveal themselves as more about the exercise of power than about public health.

Planning for the next phase of the pandemic will also heighten concerns and conflict over civil liberties. Health policy leaders have outlined a way forward that relies on widespread testing and contact tracing as prerequisites for lifting state shutdowns. Many governors, including California's Gavin Newsom and New York's Andrew Cuomo, have expressed similar sentiments.

But think hard about the details. Testing may be mandatory. Contact tracing may mean government tracking of cellphone data. How much privacy are individuals willing to forfeit for a virus that increasingly appears to pose little danger to a large percentage of the U.S. population? We will soon learn the answer.

As a strategy, this approach is probably most viable in the workplace, where employers can compel employees to undergo testing and antibody screening. Outside the workplace, compliance will likely be low, which will allow the virus to continue to spread. As infections increase after the lockdown is lifted, many will call for restrictions to be reinstated. This will further inflame disputes. It takes little more than a basic understanding of U.S. history and human nature to know that these battles over liberty will neither be trivial nor easily quieted.

The issue of mandating face masks deserves special attention. When Gov. Cuomo announced an executive order that all New Yorkers must wear masks in public, he argued, "You don't have a right to infect me." This isn't a weak argument. The counterargument is also strong: Whose burden is it to show that a person is contagious in the first place? And if people aren't contagious, on what grounds can the government force them to wear masks? Ultimately, we may not be able to escape the "immunity passports" that Anthony Fauci, director of the National Institute of Allergy and Infectious Diseases, cited as a possibility "under certain circumstances."

Dismissing sincere concerns about civil liberties may have implications for effective coordination of future pandemic efforts. Social-distancing measures are good at slowing disease outbreaks, and the wisest course is to implement them in the least burdensome and most sustainable way possible. Unfortunately, many states have already veered sharply from this path. The coming second phase of the pandemic response affords leaders a chance to demonstrate wisdom and restraint.

The Crucial Reopening Question*
Wall Street Journal, May 21, 2020

Organizations need a plan for how to react when a customer or employee tests positive for Covid-19.

---

* https://www.wsj.com/articles/the-crucial-reopening-question-11590100302.

If reopening—and staying open—is the goal, the most important question that workplaces, schools, restaurants and retailers should be asking isn't how to maintain social distancing on their premises. Nor is it how to disinfect workspaces or whether to mandate face masks. The most important question is what they will do when an employee, customer, teacher or student tests positive for Covid-19, and what they will do if that person dies.

Thinking clearly about how to handle new infections is critical to building and maintaining public confidence in reopening efforts. If organizations bungle their responses to new infections that occur within their facilities, it will serve as an invitation for political leaders again to engage in the knee-jerk, fear-fueled policy making that led us down the road of ineffectual lockdowns in the first place.

Many organizations are asking the questions that will make reopening feasible: Can students attend in-person classes in the fall? When can our employees return to the office? How soon will clients be ready to come in? As businesses aim to attract customers, their communications largely focus on enhanced cleaning methods, social-distancing protocols and face-mask mandates for employees and customers. Assurances that they will "protect the health and safety" of employers and patrons is the theme of their messages—and usually stated explicitly.

But the novel coronavirus has so far defied all efforts at containment. Despite heavy-handed lockdowns and face-mask mandates, the virus has continued to spread in every state in the U.S., according to the Johns Hopkins Coronavirus Resource Center. In New York, Gov. Andrew Cuomo noted on May 6 that it was "shocking" to find that two-thirds of patients recently hospitalized in the state were people who were sheltering at home. "They were literally at home," he added for emphasis. How can a virus that has spread during a shutdown stop spreading when the shutdown ends? It can't, and we must plan and prepare.

The White House provided a preview of why it's so important to be prepared for Covid-19 infections, and how an organization's response can influence public perception. When the vice president's press secretary and the president's personal valet tested positive earlier this month, the media painted a picture of an administration caught off guard. The subsequent implementation of new infection-prevention protocols in the White House added to this perception. All businesses and organizations are similarly vulnerable to reactive decision-making, born out of panic during times of crisis—such as when a Covid infection or death is tied to their establishment.

Panic-driven decision-making doesn't inspire public confidence. Instead, preparing now for the inevitable increase in Covid-19 infections that will accompany reopening—and publicly articulating those plans—is what organizations must do to support sustained reopening.

As if schools, businesses and entertainment venues don't have enough to worry about, they are also up against a media eager to frame every new infection as a reason not to reopen. "It is too soon," we often hear. Not enough people are asking these same media outlets and their quoted experts exactly when a good time to reopen would be.

What, therefore, should leaders do when people connected to their organizations contract Covid-19? For universities and schools that are restarting in-person teaching, the answer may be to provide testing, make reasonable attempts at contact tracing, and support those who are quarantining while offering remote learning for those at higher risk.

For workplaces, there could be temporary transitions to remote work with cleaning crews deployed following a Covid-19 diagnosis. N95 masks could be distributed to employees, as opposed to cloth face coverings that are ineffective at preventing infection for the wearer.

All leaders should keep sight of the organizational mission that spurred them to reopen in the first place. Closing shop for an indeterminate and extendible period is the wrong answer for any organization. It appeases fear and lacks a sound scientific basis.

If done right, reopening can evolve in a way that balances the things that make life worthwhile—strong social connections, purposeful work and pursuit of personal growth—against the real human threats of the novel coronavirus. If done wrong, we'll continue struggling to find our footing, creating avoidable pain and suffering along the way, until we are finally rescued by either herd immunity or a vaccine, whichever comes first.

CHAPTER 7

My Friend Simone Gold

Mindful leadership is an invaluable quality when navigating public health crises, and the country learned this the hard way in the spring and summer of 2020. Part of being mindful is being self-aware, and this includes awareness of your own beliefs, fears, hopes, and biases.

Self-awareness also means recognizing that the world is filled with people who do not share your values and therefore may not bend to your will. In other words, public health policies are bound to fail—which is to say that they will cause harm and be ineffective—if crafted in an ideology-fueled vacuum rather than in the context of people's day-to-day lives. Public health policies must be grounded in reality.

This lack of self-awareness was on stark display in May 2020, after George Floyd was tragically killed by police officers in Minneapolis, Minnesota. While many could not resist the temptation to ensnare his death in their political beliefs about racism or "structural inequality," the reality was that he was a man who was cruelly treated by other men, and the circumstances of his death were both heartbreaking and dehumanizing.

That people were roused to express their discontent was, simply, a reflection of our humanity. But the involvement of politicians—most of whom care first and foremost about their own political survival—demonstrated a profound absence of self-awareness on the part of these political leaders. These were the same people who, by and large, had been preaching breathlessly just weeks earlier about the importance of not gathering in large groups. They and their appointed public health officials doggedly promoted lockdown policies and other restrictions to daily living. Now, they walked in close quarters with thousands and sometimes tens of thousands of protestors, expressing support for the "Black Lives Matter" movement.

Their absence of awareness led many of them to fail to appreciate how other priorities—many of which are important to public health, like employment, school, and gathering to worship—merited similar deference. The double standard was not lost on many conservatives in the country, and they fumed.

After I wrote about this in another article in the *Wall Street Journal* and called out the politicization of Covid-19 pandemic policies, things became more interesting at UCLA. In this most recent article, I took a particularly "brass-knuckles" approach to criticizing health officials and political leaders who had departed far from principles of public health. Some of my colleagues began circulating a letter that was a rebuttal to my writings and the messages I espoused, even adopting and modifying an illustration the newspaper had created for my article (an illustration by David Gothard of a man with marionette strings holding up a mask on his face). These colleagues were clearly intimidated by my message and the public traction it received.

My initial reaction when I learned of this effort was horror and trepidation; after all, I had always enjoyed positive, collaborative relationships with coworkers, and I had a reputation as a faculty member with whom people liked to work. This was evident from the multiple collaborative grant applications I had submitted and been awarded in conjunction with researchers and clinicians across a variety of fields. But now, some of my colleagues were literally working to subvert me and my message.

As the development settled in my mind, my initial reaction quickly morphed into amusement. I had clearly struck a nerve, and my colleagues who were in support of the lockdown-mandates-left-wing-politics approach to the pandemic were uncomfortable with voices that dissented from their position. But I knew that none of their efforts would discourage me from continuing to speak truths that were desperately needed in the United States at the time.

It was around this time that a friend introduced me to Dr. Simone Gold. Before meeting her, I remember admiring her courage and willingness to be vocal and stand for the ideas in which she believed. The fact that much of the public health community had interpreted the COVID pandemic as an invitation to dismiss civil liberties was not lost on her, and at that point, I was deeply grateful to hear any voice that recognized this, since nearly all physicians and scientists were silent on the matter. But she had courage, and it was inspiring.

In our first conversation by phone, it was easy to see that we shared many common views of public health, and the fact that public health measures should not be implemented without considering their implications for civil liberties. While tension between public health and individual liberties will always exist, a wise rule of thumb—abandoned during the pandemic—is that the strength of an intervention's supporting evidence and its anticipated benefits must be commensurate with the burden it places on civil liberties.

In other words, interventions grounded in uncertain evidence, such as mask mandates for healthy people (people without symptoms), are not ethically permissible. After all, nearly every randomized clinical trial of mask wearing in the community found no health benefit. Moreover, mask mandates for healthy people should also almost never be implemented because the burden they impose on civil liberties is extraordinary. A person's face is one of the most intimate parts of their body, and that makes it "off limits" to public health officials, except under very special circumstances such as an active infection. Even then, one must still consider the implications of an intervention for bodily sovereignty.

Simone, who has both a medical degree and a law degree and had practiced emergency medicine for many years, was extremely enthusiastic about health policy. She invited me and a few other doctors to speak to members of Congress in early July. In our meeting that day with Congressman Andy Biggs from Arizona and other lawmakers, we discussed COVID lockdown policies, school reopenings, and communication strategies.

It was a fun trip, and I met individuals who have become lifelong friends, like Drs. Teryn Clarke, Richard Urso, and Bob Hamilton. And while the opportunity was remarkable, our discussions with the lawmakers revealed how little clarity there was—even among conservatives—about optimal policymaking during a pandemic. I felt this reflected the complexity of the issue since it spanned multiple disciplines, including clinical medicine, public health, immunology, and epidemiology. Ultimately, though, the policy preferences of these members of Congress were the "right" ones because they would actually benefit the public.

Shortly after our return, Simone contacted me and a handful of other physicians to discuss a second trip to the Capitol. She envisioned a series of educational discussions about COVID-19 lockdown policies, school reopenings, the burden on mental health and wellness, and data supporting treatment options for COVID. It was around this time that she introduced "America's Frontline Doctors" as the name for this group of physicians.

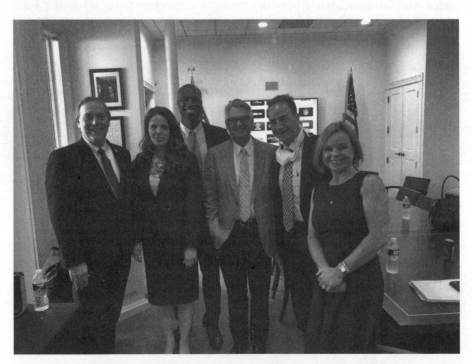

Meeting with Congressman Biggs, July 9, 2020.

This was another fun trip, and I made new friends, including Dr. Stella Immanuel. On July 27, near the end of the discussions, we assembled in front of the Supreme Court to hold a small press conference that would ultimately make history. On that hot summer day in Washington, DC, I remember enjoying the energy of the day, surrounded by other free-thinking physicians who valued good health and freedom. I also remember holding a mask in my hand while walking outside just to avoid inciting conflicts with passersby that might create a distraction from our work, as mask mandates outdoors were active at that time and COVID fear in the DC community ran deep.

When the discussion in front of the Supreme Court started, I was actually standing off to the side, talking with an angry passerby and her friend about school reopenings. She was a teacher and spoke to me about how afraid she was that she would catch COVID and die if schools were reopened, and how our group was reckless for advocating for such a position. She gave me reason after reason for why there was just no conceivable way that kids could return to school.

I listened politely, though I was smiling inside. One of the things that changed after working with Christopher is the fact that I find humor in so much more of life now, even in disagreements. I possess a greater appreciation for the unspoken beliefs and preferences that motivate people's positions, and though it probably sounds odd, this new perspective makes it possible to disagree with people while enjoying the beauty of their humanity —and being amused by the stories they are telling themselves.

Eventually, I rejoined the group of doctors on the Supreme Court steps. A handful of people had stopped by to listen, but the crowd was small and probably no more than about 20 or 30 people. When it was my turn to speak, I shared a simple message. While I personally hadn't reviewed many studies of hydroxychloroquine use in early treatment— that is to say, while patients are still at home and before they are hospitalized—it seemed terribly irrational to dismiss it at this point when some physicians reported positive outcomes with its use. And that was basically all I said.

I flew back to Los Angeles that Monday evening. The next morning, Brianna mentioned that she was receiving many messages on social media from friends asking how we were doing, worried about our welfare, and referencing a video that had gone viral. This was news to me. As I sat down at my computer to investigate, I learned that the Supreme Court event was being covered by major news outlets, that President Trump had tweeted out a video of the press conference, and that we had apparently made many, many political leaders, media personalities, and health officials upset.

I had never received this type of attention before, and it was jarring. It represented a point of no return. Brianna and I talked it through. I was worried about how my colleagues would treat me, and I also worried that this development could jeopardize my research funding. Finding ourselves in the middle of intense national controversy, we also worried about our safety.

But ultimately, we decided that we could not walk away from doing the right thing, no matter how difficult the circumstances or staunch the opposition. Our tenets of truth, justice, and human sovereignty were unraveling right in front of us, and the world desperately needed leadership free from the dark motivations of fear, greed, and control.

While we were not eager to have me or our family become a flashpoint for national controversy, we knew that more important than living safely in obscurity was being able to tell our children in 20 years that we stood firmly on the side of freedom, truth, and love. So, we made up our minds to see it through, placed our fate in God's hands, and ventured off on our Tuesday date later that morning . . . but both of us sensed that something had changed about the direction of our lives forever.

The Coronavirus Credibility Gap*
Wall Street Journal, July 1, 2020

Politicians and experts sow distrust with double standards on protests and dissembling about masks.

---

* https://www.wsj.com/articles/the-coronavirus-credibility-gap-11593645643?mod=searchresults&page=1&pos=1.

The American public is fractured over policy responses to Covid-19. That rift is most visible in debates about masks and new rounds of shutdowns. Such disputes are common in a country as diverse and opinionated as America. But political leaders and health officials have sown distrust by politicizing the pandemic response.

Political leaders and health officials have often invoked "science" to justify decisions manifestly guided by their personal preferences. That costs them credibility. Restoring public confidence will require acknowledging their role in politicizing the pandemic, yielding to accommodations and sensible alternatives in the areas of greatest controversy, and focusing on the widely supported goal of not overwhelming hospitals, rather than less meaningful metrics such as increases in Covid-19 cases.

One of the earliest signs of politicization was the broad animus directed at protesters who objected to the lockdowns. In a country where liberty and free expression are as fundamental as air and water, it is remarkable how casually political leaders and health officials disparaged and banned their activities—and even targeted protesters for prosecution. Politics was also at play when New York Mayor Bill de Blasio ordered police in Brooklyn to break up a crowd of mourners who gathered for a Hasidic Jewish funeral, warning that their actions were "unacceptable" and threatening to arrest them.

Contrast this with the approach that many of the same political leaders and public-health experts took toward the protests catalyzed by George Floyd's killing. These protesters were neither maligned nor targeted with fines and arrests based on social distancing or mask mandates. They were often joined in the streets by politicians such as Los Angeles Mayor Eric Garcetti and New Jersey Gov. Phil Murphy.

The double standard in treatment was political. All these public gatherings were led by people expressing sincerely held beliefs that they felt outweighed the risk of Covid-19 transmission. Protecting such expression, regardless of viewpoint, is fundamental to the integrity of a democracy. Instead, politicians played favorites with this core American tenet.

Medical experts have also lost the empathy that previously characterized their approach to public health. Many illnesses spread as a result of personal decisions and behavior. The contemporary consensus in the medical community has been to acknowledge—without judgment—that preferences and circumstances of individuals vary. This has been true even when individual decisions affect the health of others. This is why public-health experts advocate pre-exposure prophylaxis antiretrovirals for HIV prevention, needle-exchange programs for drug users, and, in the U.K., e-cigarettes for smoking cessation.

But this wisdom hasn't been afforded to the Covid-19 pandemic. There is little accommodation for people who avoid masks because of difficulty breathing, claustrophobia or the belief that one's face shouldn't be subject to public policing. Some medical ethicists have suggested that if ventilators are in short supply, patients who religiously used masks and adhered to social distancing should receive priority—rationing medical care to punish noncompliance.

Further corroding public trust was health officials' reversal about wearing masks. In February, they discouraged their use and told the public there was no evidence they were effective. Yet when questioned by Rep. David McKinley (R., W.Va.) on June 23, Anthony Fauci claimed the initial guidance was motivated by concerns about medical supply shortages—not doubts about mask effectiveness. No wonder many Americans don't trust the calls to wear masks.

If political leaders and health experts want to restore their credibility and the public's confidence, they need to begin by acknowledging that politics rather than science has influenced important public-health decisions and by making accommodations for dissenting perspectives. Alternatives to masks, for instance, include physical distancing and using face shields while indoors.

And while there is more to learn about immunity, there has not been a single confirmed case of reinfection among the 10 million cases of Covid-19 world-wide, according to a May report in the Journal of the American Medical Association. Until the data say otherwise, people who have recovered from Covid-19 should be exempt from restrictions.

The most important step political leaders and health officials can take is to base their decisions on hospital capacity, rather than case counts, which inevitably will continue to increase among low-risk young people. Policing of social distance and restrictions on personal, educational and business activities are fueling culture wars. Focusing on the goal of not overwhelming hospitals is sensible and less vulnerable to politicization—so long as the data are publicly available for independent analysis. Hospitals often run near capacity to maximize profits, so the promises made during shutdowns to increase capacity need to be fulfilled—or capacity will become a political weapon.

Since citizens are already opting out of high-risk activities they want to avoid, let them enter bars, enjoy the beach, exercise at the gym, and learn in school if they choose. The government should intervene with mandates and closures only if regional hospital capacity requires it, while being transparent about bed availability, illness severity of hospitalized patients, and efforts to increase treatment capacity, including the supply of promising medications such as remdesivir and dexamethasone.

These steps would make the struggle against Covid-19 more sustainable and less politicized. Less petty squabbling and wasting of resources would mean more attention for strategies to protect the most vulnerable Americans.

Transcript of Supreme Court Speech[*]
July 28, 2020

---

* "America's Frontline Doctors SCOTUS Press Conference Transcript," Rev.com, July 27, 2020,#https://www.rev.com/blog/transcripts/americas-frontline-doctors-scotus-press-conference-transcript.

Dr. Joe Ladapo: (33:27)
Sure thing. I'm Dr. Joe. Ladapo. I'm a physician at UCLA and I'm a clinical researcher also. And I'm speaking for myself and not on behalf of UCLA. So I want to say that I'm thinking of the people who are behind the screens that are watching what you guys were broadcasting. And I want to share with you because there's so much controversy and the atmosphere is so full of conflict right now that what this group of doctors is trying to do fundamentally, is really to bring more light to this conversation about how we manage Covid-19 and the huge challenge. And that's what this is ultimately about. And bringing light to something means thinking more about trade offs, about one of my colleagues said on unintended consequences. And I actually think that's not even the right word, the right word is unanticipated consequences. Really thinking about the implications of the decisions we're making in this really, really extraordinary time that we're in.

Dr. Joe Ladapo: (34:45)
So, I'm sure people are listening to some of the discussion about hydroxychloroquine and wondering, what are these doctors talking about? And, these are doctors that take care of patients, board certified, med school, great med schools, all of that. How could they possibly be saying this? I watch CNN and NBC, and they don't say anything about this. And that's actually, that's the point. There are issues that are moral issues, that really there should be a singular voice. So for me, issues related to whether people are treated differently based on their sex or race, or their sexual orientation. I personally think those are moral issues and there's only one position on those. But Covid-19 is not a moral issue. Covid-19 is a challenging, complex issue that we benefit from having multiple perspectives on. So it's not good for the American people when everyone is hearing one perspective on the main stations. There's no way that's going to service. So, the perspective most people have been hearing is that hydroxychloroquine doesn't

work. That's the perspective that most people have been hearing on the mainstream television.

Dr. Joe Ladapo: (36:03)
That's the perspective that most people have been hearing on the mainstream television, and I believe that perspective too, until I started talking to doctors who would look more closely than some of the physicians behind me here, who would look more closely at the data and at the studies.

Dr. Joe Ladapo: (36:17)
So it is a fact that several randomized trials have come out so far, that's our highest level of evidence, and have shown that hydroxychloroquine... Their findings have generally been that there's no significant effect on health benefit. So, that's a fact, that the randomized control trials have come out... So far that have come out. In fact, there were two or three big ones that came out over the last two weeks, [inaudible 00:36:44] Internal Medicine, New England Journal of Medicine, and I think one other journal.

Dr. Joe Ladapo: (36:49)
It is also a fact that there have been several observational studies. These are just not randomized controlled trials, but patients who are getting treated with this medication that have found that hydroxy-chloroquine improves outcomes. So both of those things are true. There's evidence against it and there's evidence for it. It is also a fact that we are in an extraordinarily challenging time. Given those considerations, how can the right answer be to limit physician's use of the medication? That can't possibly be the right answer. And when you consider that this medication before Covid-19 had been used for decades, by patients with rheumatoid arthritis, by patients with lupus, by patients with other conditions, by patients who were

traveling to West Africa and needed malaria prophylaxis, we've been using it for a long time, but all of a sudden it's elevated to this area of looking like some poisonous drug. That just doesn't make sense.

Dr. Joe Ladapo: (37:59)

Then when you add onto that the fact that we've had two of the biggest journals in the world, New England Journal of Medicine, and Lancet, as my colleagues say, retract studies that found, interestingly, that hydroxychloroquine harmed patients. Both of these studies. They had to retract these studies, which really is unheard of. That should raise everyone's concern about what is going on. At the very least, we can live in a world where there are differences of opinion about the effectiveness of hydroxychloroquine, but still allow more data to come, still allow physicians who feel like they have expertise with it use that medication, and still talk, and learn, and get better at helping people with Covid-19.

Dr. Joe Ladapo: (38:50)

So why we're not there is not good. It doesn't make sense, and we need to get out of there.

CHAPTER 8

Public Health's Worst Pandemic Decisions

Most of us recognize that in order to make the best decisions possible, we have to consider all relevant information we have at our disposal. This is true for decisions as simple as whether to order steak or fish at dinner with a spouse, when we might consider our dietary preferences, menu prices, and the restaurant's reputed strengths, or as complex as where to buy a house, when we might consider neighborhood safety, the quality of nearby schools and stores, and the number of children we foresee in our future.

The equivalent of this approach to decision making in public health is often referred to as a "health impact assessment." While I don't encourage uncritical acceptance of definitions put forth by parties with a vested interest in the relevant subject area, the World Health Organization's (WHO) definition of health impact assessments is reliable. (NB: Two good reasons to be mindful about definitions—particularly if they relate to pandemics—include the WHO's political decision in November 2020 to alter the definition of "herd immunity" to exclude natural infection, which they later reversed, and the CDC's removal in September 2021 of the term *immunity* from their definition of *vaccine*.)

The WHO states that a health impact assessment is a "combination of procedures, methods and tools by which a policy, program or project may be judged as to its potential effects on the health of a population, and the distribution of those effects within the population." The International Association for Impact Assessment, which has collaborated with the WHO, goes on to add that this assessment should include the "unintended" effects of a policy.

The fact that the public health community was intimately aware of "health impact assessments" as a tool for decision making is half of the reason their broad support of school closures was so appalling. The other half is the fact that the public health community has long recognized the strong relationship between education and health. I will expand on the second half before turning back to the first.

Decades of research have shown a positive correlation between education and health. The relationship has been documented across different countries and over different time periods, and while correlation does not equal causation, studies that can be used to infer causation have also found a positive relationship between education and health. In short, while questions remain—for example, Do the effects of education on health vary by how good a school is or what educational topics are taught?—it is widely recognized in public health that education is an important contributor to health.

A properly conducted health impact assessment of school closures in spring 2020 would have shown uncertain health benefits to children, given data that were already available about the extremely low risk of significant harm to children from COVID-19 and uncertainty about the role that schools played in community transmission. This same health impact assessment would also have projected a risk of adverse effects from school closures on children and adolescents—and subsequently, on their present and future health. The risk would have been uncertain because the duration of school closures was still unknown.

That would have been the assessment very early in the pandemic. By the fall of 2020, when it was time for the next school year to start, we already had data from other countries, like Sweden, indicating that keeping schools open was safe for children and that schools did not appear to substantially contribute to transmission. In other words, any potential benefits were very near zero.

Meanwhile, the harms associated with school closures were coming sharply into focus: children from all walks of life were struggling with remote "learning," low-income families in particular were being left behind, and some large school districts, such as Los Angeles Unified School District, were losing track of large numbers of previously enrolled children who never showed up for remote learning.

There were also unintended consequences to worry about. What were the risks of placing children in front of computer screens for long periods of time? Prior research had led pediatricians to recommend against doing this very thing for years. What about the effects of school closures on the family? Many parents were forced to change or even forgo their work schedules in order to help their children with remote learning, and this seemed to affect women more than men. And what about the effects of decreased social interaction on child development? Research and common sense argued strongly for the importance of social interaction for normal development.

A health impact assessment performed in the weeks leading up to the fall 2020 school year would therefore have shown that school closures were extraordinarily likely to be harmful to children and society. The fact that many members of the public health community continued to lend support for prolonged school closures despite this fact is one of the most heartbreaking aspects of the pandemic. The health and wellness of children were carelessly cast aside when it would have been so simple to prioritize.

If there were only two pieces of advice I could share with future generations about public health decision making during a pandemic, the first would be to avoid closing schools. The only time this course of action would be justified is when the benefits to kids *actually* outweigh the harms. This was *never* the case—not at one single point—during the COVID-19 pandemic in the United States.

By March 2020, when lockdown frenzy set in, we already knew from Wuhan that children were almost universally unharmed by COVID-19.

Later, we would learn that children with preexisting conditions, such as diabetes or chronic lung disease, were at increased risk compared to children who were healthy. But those same data would show that their risk from COVID-19 was still far, far lower than the risk faced by adults.

The second piece of advice I would share with future generations is to avoid forcing people to wear face masks. Of all the pandemic policies that callously restricted civil liberties—and there were many—the mask mandates were the most divisive and demoralizing, and they did the most to perpetuate an atmosphere of fear. For the data-based reason for why this also proved to be an ineffective policy, I refer readers to *Unmasked: The Global Failure of COVID Mask Mandates* by Ian Miller. For a shorter overview, I wrote a piece in the *Wall Street Journal* on October 29. 2020.

"Wearing a mask was no problem for me," you say? Good for you and for others who felt similarly. But millions of your fellow Americans felt strongly that forcing them to place something over their mouth and nose, obstructing their faces and impeding their ability to breathe clearly, crossed a line. It infringed on their personal sovereignty and caused health concerns, and the coercion was demoralizing. To make matters worse, everywhere from grocery stores to airplanes, mask mandates fueled an unimaginable amount of angst, conflict, and division throughout the United States. They are the poster children for terrible public health policy.

In our own household, Brianna and I naturally and independently arrived at a "not a snowball's chance in hell" position on mask wearing for our kids. Los Angeles Unified School District was starting the 2020–2021 year with remote learning anyway, so the issue was moot as far as school went. But in terms of how to navigate remote learning, Brianna and I had different ideas—but fortunately, she helped me see the light.

I was deeply worried about the boys falling behind, since they had been out of school since March, and I thought that remote learning might be better than whatever alternative we could put together. "No way, baby," Brianna told me. "It is far more important that we protect their emotional health and keep their light protected from all the fear and darkness. They can always learn what they miss in school. Right now, it's much more important that we keep their little spirits safe."

I was initially resistant, but, my goodness, she was right. Fortunately, it did not take too long for me to realize it. As the first day of the school year approached, I contacted our oldest son's teacher to schedule a virtual meeting. I explained that the boys' schedule and my work schedule would not allow us to easily participate in the remote learning curriculum live. She fortunately agreed to allow us to continue doing lessons on our own time and submit them electronically.

"Phew," I thought with relief. The boys would be able to continue their schedule of going to the park in the mornings and doing schoolwork in the afternoon, and we didn't have to fight with the teacher to accommodate this. For my middle son, he would have started transitional kindergarten that fall, but we chose to not enroll him, like many other Los Angeles parents during the pandemic. We bought him some good kindergarten workbooks and opted to teach him alongside his older brother. Our toddler was too young for school anyway, so there was no issue there. Fortunately, we also found a babysitter who was studying to be an elementary school teacher, so was perfectly equipped to help us homeschool the boys.

On our Tuesday brunch dates around this time, Brianna and I would often discuss our frustration with the Los Angeles school system and California's pandemic management. These conversations spurred me to write an article in the *Wall Street Journal* that targeted the malignancy of forced masking without strong evidence of health benefits and forced school closures despite the evidence they were causing kids harm. We were both exasperated with the callousness and absurdity of harmful, divisive restrictions with no end in sight, particularly the continued closure of Los Angeles schools.

This article was published on August 3, 2020, and was somewhat fiery in tone. I followed it up with a more conciliatory, reflective article published in the *Wall Street Journal* on September 16, 2020, that rehashed some of the same issues but described a path forward for states to start living with the virus in a sustainable manner.

Editors at the *Wall Street Journal* produced art for the August article that was particularly poignant. In a remake of *The Scream* by Norwegian

artist Edvard Munch in 1893, the picture displayed mask-wearing report-
ers whose faces were riddled with anxiety and dread as they covered the
pandemic. In the background stood a politician holding a mask, though
the reader is left to decide whether he is taking it off to speak or putting
it on for the cameras. You can guess which I think is correct.

The messages in these articles would have been considered bread-
and-butter public health in the past: education of children is important, avoid divisive policies with little or no proven benefit, avoid using
fear as a communication strategy, and consider both benefits and costs
associated with policies. But thanks to the dearth of competent public
health leadership, coupled with Dr. Anthony Fauci's infatuation with
the limelight and with seeding the American consciousness with fear,
there were few public health experts who were voicing perspectives similar to mine.

Brianna and I felt compelled to fill the void. And while doors were
closing at UCLA in terms of my relationship with the institution's leaders
and some of my colleagues, new doors were opening, including one that
would lead to a meeting with President Trump.

Fear and Loathing in Covid America[*]
Wall Street Journal, August 3, 2020

*Public panic and media scorn are shutting down important debates
about how to tackle the virus.*

The fear surrounding Covid-19, combined with the media's judgmental portrayal of new coronavirus cases as failures of political
leadership and citizen morality, are backing policy makers into a
corner and seeding social turmoil. Rising case numbers are the
expected result of basic, powerful human desires to participate
in life. Rather than acknowledge this, politicians are allowing
fear to fuel poor policy decisions. A course correction will require

---

[*] https://www.wsj.com/articles/fear-and-loathing-in-covid-america-11596470084.

empowering Americans to prevent illness and absolving ourselves from the prevailing narrative.

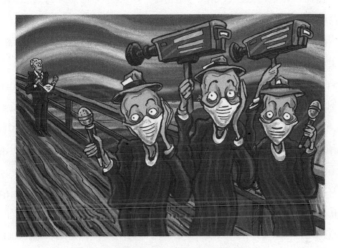

Illustration: Chad Crowe

The profound shift in public-policy goals from March to the present is a powerful demonstration of the effects of public fear and a judgmental narrative from the press. In March, Americans understood that Mother Nature can sometimes be unforgiving in matters of life and death. There was broad public support for the prudent goals of preventing hospitals from being overwhelmed and buying scientists time to develop therapies.

But as those goals were accomplished, fear stoked by the press gave birth to the dogma that preventing Covid-19 cases isn't an issue only of health but of morality—even if prevention comes at the cost of livelihoods and futures, or increases poverty and domestic violence, or sacrifices children's educational and emotional well-being. Statewide shutdowns were extended, and states with case increases were deemed to have incompetent leaders and citizens who were behaving "selfishly" and "not following rules."

The problem with public-health strategies born of fear and disdain is that they create unrealistic expectations and smother dissent. The country has shifted from a period of public unity and cooperation in March to one of blame and opprobrium. Approaches to managing the pandemic that fall outside mainstream thought are shut down. States become willing to make trade-offs that would have been unthinkable in saner times.

An example is the use of masks. As a result of energetic scientific inquiry, there is now evidence that reducing the transmission of respiratory droplets with masks is associated with reductions in Covid-19 transmission, primarily when indoors. But before the pandemic, at least 10 randomized clinical trials yielded mixed results on community masking for influenza, with several studies showing no effects on transmission.

It is reasonable to suggest that these clinical trials may not be applicable to the current circumstances, given the chance of Covid-19 transmission from those without symptoms and variation in mask compliance. But the minimal attention these trials received is an example of how fear has eroded reason and curiosity and replaced these virtues with whatever is most expedient.

Los Angeles has had a mask mandate in place for people outside their homes since May. Gov. Gavin Newsom issued a similar mandate for the state of California in June. While these mandates have likely decreased Covid-19 transmission, the 2,400 new cases Los Angeles County averaged daily over the past week show that masks aren't the cure-all the media often presents them as.

If the counterargument is that those in Los Angeles aren't wearing masks while walking down the street or at the beach, consider that indoor—not outdoor—transmission is the driver of the pandemic. One contact tracing study in China involving 318 outbreaks and 1,245 cases of Covid-19 identified only a single incident of outdoor transmission. This basic evidence didn't stop District of Columbia officials from threatening $1,000 fines on people not wearing masks outdoors. Policies like this are about politicians flexing power and looking tough; they are not about public health.

Then there's the debate about reopening schools. Because of the moral deference given to preventing Covid-19 transmission, it is now possible for school districts to deprive children casually—and indefinitely—of an environment that nurtures their educational, social and emotional development, all of which affects long-term health, income and well-being. This injury is compounded by data from multiple countries that show children are the least likely to be harmed by the virus. Concerns about transmission from students to teachers, parents and vulnerable family members are valid. But the toxic political environment has choked off any earnest discussion about solutions that could satisfy all these concerns.

A path to breaking the grip of fear on society is through empowerment. Though the Centers for Disease Control and Prevention's guidance about masks focuses on protecting others and is cast in the language of altruism, it is doing little to empower citizens. Telling people their fate lies in the hands of others leaves them feeling powerless and frustrated when others don't comply.

One way to empower people would be resolving the shortage of personal protective equipment and providing older Americans, other vulnerable populations and anyone else who wants it with easy access to the tools that are reducing infection risk in health-care workers, such as medical masks and face shields. Communicating the role of good nutrition, exercise and stress reduction—all things we can control—as facilitators of immune function would also increase personal empowerment and reduce fear.

Other critical steps include increasing the supply of effective therapies, improving communication about mortality risk—which is low for most people—and increasing access to rapid testing for those in contact with vulnerable populations.

And what should be done about the media and public derision that is haunting leaders and vexing citizens? Everyone needs simply to stop participating. It is a terrible way to implement public-health interventions, and it sows conflict and diminishes morale. We all need to get off this treadmill.

How to Live with Covid, Not for It[*]
Wall Street Journal, September 16, 2020

If reason finally prevails over panic, policy makers will reopen schools and focus on the vulnerable.

The battle against Covid-19 is entering a new phase, and the choice for society is whether to live with the virus or to live for it. This new phase has been marked by four developments: Many states have weathered post-shutdown outbreaks and case counts are falling; the percentage of Americans saying the pandemic is worsening peaked in July and is trending down, according to Gallup polling; the culture wars over lockdowns and distancing mandates are cooling; and inexpensive rapid testing and a vaccine will soon be available widely. These developments create an atmosphere of possibility—and an opportunity to pivot away from the fear-fueled policy-making that has characterized the pandemic.

Policies forged in fear and panic have wrought tremendous damage in exchange for benefits that were attainable at a much lower cost. Over the past six months, we have managed to sow vicious conflict over health mandates among people who would otherwise be cordial; erode age-old social customs, like visible smiles and human touch, which are critical to social cohesion and personal well-being; and condemn millions of Americans to financial instability, depression and even domestic violence.

The collective goal of this new phase should be to avoid repeating the mistakes of the past. When faced in March with the choice between imposing limited shutdowns to buy hospitals time and increase capacity, and enormous, indefinite shutdowns that ignored societal and economic costs, most political leaders chose the latter. When faced in May and June with the choice between embracing policies that balanced Covid-19 prevention with the activities that

---

[*] https://www.wsj.com/articles/how-to-live-with-covid-not-for-it-11600271921.

give life meaning and policies that sowed distrust and stirred fierce passions over civil liberties, most political leaders chose the latter. We have the opportunity to choose differently this time.

Some signs point toward institutions shifting away from fear-fueled decision making. The Centers for Disease Control and Prevention issued guidance last month that contacts of persons with Covid-19 "do not necessarily" need testing if they are asymptomatic. Early testing among those infected with the virus may yield false negatives, and testing vulnerable adults and their contacts is far more valuable than testing healthy young adults. The CDC now recommends focusing tests where they are likely to yield the greatest public-health benefits.

The good sense of this recommendation is so plain, it is almost stupefying. Where is the controversy in placing disproportionate energy and attention on populations that are disproportionately at risk for harm from Covid-19? Residents of nursing homes and other long-term care facilities—who represent less than 1% of the U.S. population—have comprised nearly half of deaths from Covid-19. A recent study in Annals of Internal Medicine reported that the infection fatality rate in noninstitutionalized persons under 40 was 0.01%, compared with 1.7% among people older than 60—a nearly 200-fold difference. Sensible policies focus special attention on populations facing the greatest harm.

The criticism the CDC has received underscores the determination of too many leaders and health officials to continue choosing fear-fueled policy-making. Consider the facts: The average Covid-19 transmission rate to close contacts is roughly 10% or 15%. The actual number of infections may be six to 24 times the number of reported cases, according to a July study in JAMA Internal Medicine. It would be impossible to close the wide gap between detected and undetected cases without resort to authoritarianism. It's clear that testing low-risk contacts is a low-value activity.

But critics of the CDC's new recommendation subscribe to the belief—knowingly or not—that all attempts to stop Covid-19 transmission are worthwhile, no matter how small the benefit or how high the cost. Increased public recognition of—and scientific support for—sensible policies will steer us away from destructive decisions fueled by fear.

There is also an opportunity to revisit decisions about schooling made by educational institutions at every level. College administrators in Ohio are expending substantial energy trying to stop young people from socializing; high schools in Georgia are being pushed toward closure due to mass quarantining; and intricate plans are being drafted for young children—for whom the virus is less harmful than seasonal influenza—in districts such as Los Angeles.

Placing disproportionate focus on Covid-19 transmission in low-risk populations leads to unwise decisions that do more harm than good. A wiser investment would focus on protecting vulnerable populations, including older teachers, family members and essential employees, by directing testing and personal protective equipment to them and their close contacts. Early outpatient therapies for Covid-19 may also prevent serious illness in these populations, as described in a recent American Journal of Medicine article.

The CDC's quarantine guidelines for healthy, low-risk students should be revisited in light of the outsize effect quarantines have on their educational experience—and the possibility of perpetual quarantining for exposed students if testing is performed frequently. University policies for Covid-19 prevention also have an edge of cruelty: Many of these administrators suspending students "caught" socializing would have been doing the same 30 or 40 years ago.

The point of life is living, and everyone is better off with policies that focus on protecting the most vulnerable populations. That doesn't take universal rapid testing or never-ending mandates. It requires only abandoning fear, being sensible about who is targeted for testing and protections, expanding treatment capacity and therapies—and choosing to live with the virus, rather than to live for it.

Masks Are a Distraction From the Pandemic Reality*
Wall Street Journal, October 28, 2020

Viruses inevitably spread, and authorities have oversold face coverings as a preventive measure.

A hallmark of Covid-19 pandemic policy has been the failure of political leaders and health officials to anticipate the unintended consequences of their actions. This tendency has haunted many decisions, from lockdowns that triggered enormous unemployment and increased alcohol and drug abuse, to school closures that are widening educational disparities between rich and poor families. Mask mandates may also have unintended consequences that outweigh the benefits.

First, consider how the debate has evolved and the underlying scientific evidence. Several randomized trials of community or household masking have been completed. Most have shown that wearing a mask has little or no effect on respiratory virus transmission, according to a review published earlier this year in Emerging Infectious Diseases, the Centers for Disease Control and Prevention's journal. In March, when Anthony Fauci said, "wearing a mask might make people feel a little bit better" but "it's not providing the perfect protection that people think it is," his statement reflected scientific consensus, and was consistent with the World Health Organization's guidance.

Almost overnight, the recommendations flipped. The reason? The risk of asymptomatic transmission. Health officials said mask mandates were now not only reasonable but critical. This is a weak rationale, given that presymptomatic spread of respiratory viruses isn't a novel phenomenon in public health. Asymptomatic cases of influenza occur in up to a third of patients, according to a 2016 report in Emerging Infectious Diseases, and even more patients had

* https://www.wsj.com/articles/masks-are-a-distraction-from-the-pandemic-reality-11603927026.

mild cases that are never diagnosed. Asymptomatic or mild cases appear to contribute more to Covid-19 transmission, but this happens in flu cases, too, though no one has called for mask mandates during flu season.

The public assumes that research performed since the beginning of the pandemic supports mask mandates. Policy makers and the media point to low-quality evidence, such as a study of Covid-19 positive hairstylists in Missouri or a Georgia summer camp with an outbreak. These anecdotes, while valuable, tell us nothing about the experience of other hairdressers or other summer camps that adopted similar or different masking practices. Also low-quality evidence: Videos of droplets spreading through air as people talk, a well-intended line of research that has stoked fears about regular human interactions.

Rather, the highest-quality evidence so far is studies like the one published in June in Health Affairs, which found that U.S. states instituting mask mandates had a 2% reduction in growth rates of Covid-19 compared with states without these mandates. Because respiratory virus spread is exponential, modest reductions can translate into large differences over time. But these shifts in trajectory are distinct from the notion that mandating masks will bring the pandemic to an end. Based on evidence around the world, it should be clear that mask mandates won't extinguish the virus.

The most reasonable conclusion from the available scientific evidence is that community mask mandates have—at most—a small effect on the course of the pandemic. But you wouldn't know that from watching cable news or sitting next to a mother being forced off an airplane because her small children aren't able to keep a mask on.

While mask-wearing has often been invoked in explanations for rising or falling Covid-19 case counts, the reality is that these trends reflect a basic human need to interact with one another. Claims that low mask compliance is responsible for rising case counts are also not supported by Gallup data, which show that the percentage of Americans reporting wearing masks has been high and relatively stable since June. Health officials and political leaders have assigned mask mandates a gravity unsupported by empirical research.

On even shakier scientific ground is the promotion of mask use outdoors. One contact-tracing study identified only a single incident of outdoor transmission among 318 outbreaks. Even the Rose Garden nomination ceremony for Justice Amy Coney Barrett, which the media giddily labeled a "superspreader" event, likely wasn't; transmission more likely occurred during indoor gatherings associated with the ceremony.

By paying outsize and scientifically unjustified attention to masking, mask mandates have the unintended consequence of delaying public acceptance of the unavoidable truth. In countries with active community transmission and no herd immunity, nothing short of inhumane lockdowns can stop the spread of Covid-19, so the most sensible and sustainable path forward is to learn to live with the virus.

Shifting focus away from mask mandates and toward the reality of respiratory viral spread will free up time and resources to protect the most vulnerable Americans. There is strong evidence that treating patients early in outpatient settings can be effective, as outlined in a recent *American Journal of Medicine* paper, but these treatments are underused. Identifying effective treatments for hospitalized patients with Covid-19 is essential, but preventing severe illness before hospitalization will save more lives.

Until the reality of viral spread in the U.S.—with or without mask mandates—is accepted, political leaders will continue to feel justified in keeping schools and businesses closed, robbing young people of the opportunity to invest in their futures, and restricting activities that make life worthwhile. Policy makers ought to move forward with more wisdom and sensibility to mitigate avoidable costs to human life and well-being.

CHAPTER 9

Meeting President Trump

Fortune led me to meet President Trump toward the end of August 2020. Dr. Scott Atlas invited me and a few other individuals to the White House while he was serving as a special advisor to the president and a member of the White House Coronavirus Task Force. I had never met Scott before, but we had spoken by phone a few times during the pandemic. Our earliest conversations were about reopening schools.

I admired Scott's willingness to stick to data-based and common-sense recommendations about pandemic health policy—a rarity at the time. For his trouble, he earned the ire of nearly the entire scientific community, which was intent on maintaining the harshest pandemic policies, despite the lack of supporting evidence. Scott seemed to be under constant assault from physicians, health officials, and political leaders.

Though Scott was ultimately proven to be correct on every assessment he made about COVID-19 health risks and pandemic management, the news media would give no quarter. To them, he was not only guilty of the sin of disagreement with the mainstream narrative (of which I was also guilty), but the cardinal sin of working with Trump.

Scott invited me and Drs. Jay Bhattacharya, Martin Kulldorff, and Cody Meissner to the White House for a meeting with President Trump regarding pandemic policy, especially lockdowns and reopening schools. When Scott and I spoke prior to the meeting, he told me that he wanted the president to hear from experts outside of those with whom he usually communicated so he could see that there were, indeed, reputable scientists who disagreed with how most health officials were managing the pandemic.

As Scott described in his book *A Plague Upon Our House*, this meeting was almost canceled at the last minute because of political opposition, but fortunately, Scott pushed it through. Because I purchased the audiobook, I had no idea that he included a picture of our meeting in the hardcover version of his book until a stranger told me. The sight of the picture and the caption underneath it still brings a warm smile to my face.

The experience of sitting in the Oval Office was amazing. I felt as though I were placing my fingers right on the pulse of history. I thought of the presidents who had previously sat there, the guests with whom they had met, and the conversations and decisions that room had witnessed. I was truly overwhelmed and remember taking deep breaths to help me calm. It was also surreal to meet President Trump, who was previously known to me only through news stories.

We had a productive conversation with President Trump. It was clear that he intuitively understood that the cure was worse than the disease in terms of the societal costs associated with the pandemic measures Dr. Fauci and his delegates in the scientific community were imposing upon the U.S. population. We discussed school closures, pandemic restrictions, and how health officials and the media were misinterpreting—and sometimes misrepresenting—what we had learned about the epidemiology of the coronavirus.

I was also very fortunate to be in the presence of remarkable scientific minds. Jay and I had met during my job search in 2016 when I interviewed at Stanford, as our family sought a new home that would be better for Brianna's migraines. It was great to see him again, as we had bonded over email exchanges and phone calls during the pandemic. He is an incredibly kind guy and very, very smart. He and Martin—whom I hadn't previously met—were two authors of the Great Barrington Deceleration, and it was a pleasure to meet them in person, too. It was also a treat to meet Cody, whom I've grown to know as a kind, gentle man with a wealth of experience in immunology and vaccine policy.

As Scott describes in his book, our meeting with President Trump ended up running much longer than planned. It was a "hit" both because of the meaningful subjects we covered and because all five of us had a genuinely nice time together. That evening, we met for dinner and drinks at a local restaurant and talked more about the meeting and the direction the country was headed in, in terms of COVID-19 policies and practices. It really was a fun trip, and I am immensely grateful to Scott for inviting me.

Before the meeting, Scott suggested that I avoid discussing treatments for COVID-19 with President Trump. "No problem," I responded. My sense was that Scott wanted to avoid anything that encouraged President Trump to consider mentioning hydroxychloroquine in press conferences because of concern about negative media responses.

But treatment is an important part of a sustainable and effective public health strategy and was largely ignored and frequently belittled during the pandemic's first two years. It is likely that this decision to sideline treatment cost the lives of hundreds of thousands of Americans, and I discuss the reasons why in the next chapter.

CHAPTER 10

From Hydroxychloroquine to Fluvoxamine: Treating Patients with COVID-19

A sad chapter in the tomes of medical history is the story of how "treatment" for covid became a dirty word. How that came to be happens to be entwined with one of the main themes of this book.

A little mindfulness can go a long way, partly because cracking a door and letting some light in may make it easier to see other doors that were previously hidden. In the best-case scenario, a sequence of discovery prompted by personal exploration leads to a virtuous progression in insights and understanding. It is analogous to the adage that the first step toward a goal is often the hardest to take, but the most important.

Regarding the treatment of COVID-19 with hydroxychloroquine, more mindfulness on the part of physicians and public health officials would almost certainly have been tremendously valuable to the American people—and people all over the world. The vehement proclamations that hydroxychloroquine "doesn't work" before the answer was knowable, the vile comments hurled toward doctors who felt hydroxychloroquine was effective in their patients, and the lack of curiosity about the experience of physicians who were treating patients and reporting success were all clear indicators of a strong underlying bias against this medication.

And where did this bias come from? The short answer is politics—particularly an aversion to President Trump. It persisted because of a remarkable lack of mindfulness and self-awareness among many health professionals. Before continuing, however, I want to acknowledge all the health professionals who were unswayed by physicians loudly railing against hydroxychloroquine on TV (many of whom probably did not bother to read scientific publications about the medication themselves) and instead listened to their clinical intuition, reviewed the primary scientific papers, or called a colleague with more experience for his or her input.

Ultimately, many health professionals and individuals from the media were profoundly unable to separate their feelings about President Trump from their feelings about hydroxychloroquine, a medication that had nothing to do with him. The intensity of their aversion to him allowed many to justify to themselves a wide range of decisions they might otherwise consider unacceptable.

For example, many knowingly or unknowingly undermined their own scientific credibility just to be on the side of a pandemic issue opposite to Trump's. Think prolonged school closures or denying natural immunity. And who knows, maybe I would have been one of those "the end justifies the means" doctors had I not worked with Christopher Maher and rid myself of the fear that was compromising my judgment.

Early in the pandemic, if the goal was to save lives, then a public health strategy that included treating high-risk patients using any safe medication that had reasonable evidence of benefit would always be a wiser, more clinically sound strategy than not treating a high-risk patient at all. The reason is that there would have been little downside, a potentially large upside, and data could be collected in the meantime to clarify any uncertainty about effectiveness.

Instead, though, the public health response led by Dr. Fauci and other leaders was characterized by dogmatic statements against treatment—and their position almost certainly cost many lives. These tragic, unnecessary losses could have been averted if more physicians and public health leaders were mindful of their biases. This is why mindfulness work is so important for public health leadership, a topic I expand on in Chapter 12.

Only the Lord knows for sure whether hydroxychloroquine is a beneficial treatment for prevention and treatment of COVID-19, but I will present to you, dispassionately, the reason why I believe the answer to that question is "yes."

First, it is important to clarify that the setting in which I think hydroxychloroquine is effective is in patients who are either taking the medication for prevention of COVID-19 or taking the medication for early treatment of COVID-19, probably within the first 5 to 7 days of illness. The setting to which I am *not* referring is in patients who are hospitalized with COVID-19 or have been ill for a protracted period of time. Randomized clinical trials in this setting have been fairly high in quality, and their results, in my opinion, indicate that the medication is unlikely to be beneficial in this setting.

So what data inform effectiveness of hydroxychloroquine as prevention for or early treatment of COVID-19? This list is not exhaustive, and surely new studies will be published, which could change the balance of my decision or strengthen my opinion. But the opinion I share here is based on the studies of which I am aware.

For simplicity, I will focus on randomized clinical trials. These studies, when properly executed, are much less vulnerable to confounding than studies that do not randomize patients to treatment. It is worth noting that my friend Dr. Harvey Risch, a brilliant epidemiologist at Yale, is a strong proponent of using both randomized and nonrandomized clinical trials to inform health policy. His argument, which is based on systematic reviews that predate the pandemic (hence, the reviews are not motivated by any pandemic politics) and have been published in leading journals, is that these two study types largely lead to similar conclusions.

But in order to avoid the technical nuances of this debate, I'll stick to randomized clinical trials. I have included the PubMed reference number (PMID) of each study, when available (PubMed is a search engine maintained by the National Institutes of Health that catalogs studies in the life science and biomedical areas). Among these studies, there are

trials that used different doses of hydroxychloroquine to test its potential ability to prevent COVID-19, either as prophylaxis before people are
exposed or after they are exposed to the virus.

Focusing first on studies that use hydroxychloroquine as prophylaxis
before people are exposed, these trials include a study of 1,483 healthcare
workers published in the journal *Clinical Infectious Diseases* by Dr. Radha
Rajasingham (PMID 33068425), a study of 200 healthcare workers published in the journal *Cureus* by Dr. Fibhaa Syed (PMID 35103151), a study
of 127 healthcare workers published in the journal *PLoS One* by Dr. Jorge
Rojas-Serrano (PMID 35139097), a study of 132 healthcare workers published in the journal *JAMA Internal Medicine* by Dr. Benjamin Abella
(PMID 33001138), a study of 624 healthcare workers published in the
journal *International Journal of Infectious Diseases* by Dr. John McKinnon
(PMID 34954095), and a study of 1,360 healthcare workers (unpublished,
but results available online at ClinicalTrials.gov) led by Dr. Adrian Hernandez of Duke University.

Of these studies, five out of six of them (the studies by Rajasingham,
Rojas-Serrano, Abella, McKinnon, and Hernandez) found that patients
who received hydroxychloroquine were diagnosed with COVID-19 at a
lower rate. Sometimes this difference was very small and sometimes it
was substantial, but it was never statistically significant.

Therefore, the conclusion of each of these studies was that there
was no significant difference between the hydroxychloroquine and placebo groups, because the statistical tests we use to measure effect found
there was insufficient precision to conclude the findings were not due to
chance. Notably, the largest of these two trials (Rajasingham and Hernandez) both reported effects that were similar in magnitude.

Looking next at the studies that used hydroxychloroquine as prophylaxis after people were exposed, these trials include a study of 821 adults
published in the journal *The New England Journal of Medicine* by Dr.
David Boulware (PMID 32492293), a study of 829 adults published in
the journal *Annals of Internal Medicine* by Dr. Ruanne Barnabas (PMID
33284679), and a study of 2,314 adults published in the journal *The New
England Journal of Medicine* by Dr. Oriol Mitjà (PMID 33289973).

Of these studies, two out of three of them (the studies by Boulware and Mitjà) found that patients treated with hydroxychloroquine were diagnosed with COVID-19 at a lower rate. Again, these differences were not statistically significant. Notably, the magnitude of the estimated effect of hydroxychloroquine was similar between these two trials.

The pattern is similar for clinical trials that used hydroxychloroquine for early treatment of COVID-19 among patients who were still home and not hospitalized. Here, we have a handful of studies, including a study of 231 adults published in the journal *EClinicalMedicine* by Dr. Christine Johnston (PMID 33681731), a study of 441 adults published in the journal *JAMA Network Open* by Dr. Gilmar Reis (PMID 33885775), a study of 491 adults published in the journal *Annals of Internal Medicine* by Dr. Caleb Skipper (PMID 32673060), a study of 293 adults published in the journal *Clinical Infectious Diseases* by Dr. Oriol Mitjà (PMID 32674126), and a study of 148 adults published in the journal *Canadian Medical Association Journal Open* by Dr. Ilan Schwartz (PMID 34145052).

For patients receiving early treatment for COVID-19, the outcomes that are most important include hospitalization, which is a proxy for severe illness, and death. Of these studies, all but the study by Dr. Ilan Schwartz found that patients treated with hydroxychloroquine were hospitalized or died less often than patients who did not receive treatment. Like the prior studies, these differences were not precise enough to be considered statistically significant.

In clinical science, the way we usually deal with this type of ambiguity is with a meta-analysis. A meta-analysis combines findings from multiple studies and synthesizes them to come up with an overall effect that is usually more precise than what could have been deduced from any of the studies individually. Sometimes, when several studies find that a result is not statistically significant because they did not enroll enough patients, this result becomes statistically significant when the studies are pooled together.

Harvey Risch and I performed one early in the pandemic, along with two other colleagues, but it had limitations. For example, we combined studies of prevention with studies of treatment because so few studies were available at the time. Another limitation was that the study outcomes we used were not all uniform, but rather focused on the most severe outcome reported by the authors. Again, this adaption was a result of the limited number of studies available. We describe our findings in an article published by the *New York Daily News* on October 13, 2020. An updated meta-analysis should be done for hydroxychloroquine, since none, to the best of my knowledge, includes more recent studies.

In the absence of an up-to-date meta-analysis, my sense is that the multiple studies that have shown a trend toward improvement among study participants treated with hydroxychloroquine indicate that the medication probably has benefit for the prevention and early treatment of COVID-19. Said differently, based on the published studies, I would expect that if these trials enrolled a larger number of patients than initially planned, or achieved their enrollment goals rather than stopping enrollment early (the Surgisphere scandal falsely raised concerns about hydroxychloroquine-related adverse events and their *Lancet* publication was later retracted, but not before multiple studies terminated enrollment early), their findings would have achieved statistical significance and shown that hydroxychloroquine is effective in the prevention or early treatment of COVID-19.

For any reader who might recoil at these words, that reaction is a sure sign that you are invested in reaching a specific conclusion about the medication—and that approach to decision making does not serve the public. For readers who are elated, I admit that I have a soft spot for you because you have been underdogs during the pandemic. Nonetheless, it is important to note that studies that have not yet been published could tip the scale in the other direction (and I have undoubtedly missed some published studies in this abbreviated review).

At this point, monoclonal antibodies for treating COVID-19 are available and large pharmaceutical companies have developed oral antiviral therapies, so the question regarding hydroxychloroquine's potential effectiveness is not really clinically significant. But it is critically significant if we want to avoid making poor decisions during future pandemics and public health crises.

If a future meta-analysis shows that, in fact, hydroxychloroquine is likely to be effective for outpatients based on the randomized clinical trials that were performed, it will join the long list of decisions and recommendations advocated by the public health community that, in retrospect, sprouted from political biases rather than hard science. Included in this list are lockdowns, school closures, and community mask mandates. Should it be surprising that the scientific community, which enthusiastically cheered along these interventions but railed against hydroxychloroquine, was again incorrect? Of course not. This is the price when mindful leadership is absent in public health.

Two other medications that are likely to be effective in outpatient care for COVID-19 and had supportive evidence for effectiveness early in the pandemic are inhaled budesonide and fluvoxamine. The pattern of clinical evidence for these two medications is similar to that for hydroxychloroquine—multiple studies generally pointing in the same direction (favoring benefit), with a few finding no benefit. There are other treatments that have been advocated for by some physicians, but I am not mentioning them in this chapter because I am less familiar with the clinical studies supporting or refuting their use.

Side effects of these medications also have to be considered. Inhaled budesonide is probably the most benign of the three medications, while fluvoxamine is probably the least well-tolerated, with many patients developing nausea. Hydroxychloroquine also increases the risk of a heart rhythm problem, though this is uncommon. These risks must be considered in treatment decisions, but overall, their safety is comparable to other commonly used medications.

In terms of public health leadership, the data were sufficient early in the pandemic to recommend the use of hydroxychloroquine, inhaled budesonide, and fluvoxamine for outpatient treatment of COVID-19. The case fatality rate exceeded a startling 10 percent for older adults in the first year of the pandemic, which likely could have been avoided had these early treatment options been given fair consideration. An analysis of risks and benefits surely favored treatment, and the correct policy decision would have been to encourage treatment while aggressively enrolling patients in clinical trials to clarify uncertainty.

With millions of people testing positive during surges, the nation and the world could have had answers to any outstanding safety or efficacy questions about these medications within a matter of weeks. That was the path of fearless leadership, and I argued this point in an article published in the *Wall Street Journal* on November 24, 2020. Sadly, it was to no avail. With high probability, this leadership failure in the public health and medical community cost hundreds of thousands of lives worldwide—at least.

And finally, a discussion about treatment would not be complete without acknowledging the individuals who fought unendingly for early treatment to be provided to patients with COVID-19. Whatever the truth is in terms of the effectiveness of these treatments, their intentions were in the right place. And for their troubles, they have braved derision from the media and physician colleagues, licensing board investigations, and social medial censorship. They are heroes.

Let's All Be Honest about Hydroxychloroquine: Evidence Is More Positive Than Many in the Medical Community Admit[*]
New York Daily News, October 13, 2020

By Dr. Joseph A. Ladapo and Dr. Harvey A. Risch

Let's all be honest about hydroxychloroquine: Evidence is more positive than many in the medical community admit.

Hydroxychloroquine is ineffective and unsafe in the treatment of Covid-19: This is the belief held by millions of Americans and many healthcare professionals. After months of randomized clinical trials yielding findings that were not statistically significant, and others

---

[*] https://www.nydailynews.com/opinion/ny-oped-lets-all-be-honest-about-hydroxychloroquine-20201013
-5j5q4i23qvfuzos4jh7ztc3usa-story.html.

reporting side effects, no one could be blamed for reaching this conclusion.

But an important slice of the hydroxychloroquine data tells a different story.

Because of the medication's politicization, and the pernicious tendency for dissenting perspectives to be silenced during the pandemic, data supporting hydroxychloroquine's effectiveness have been almost inaudible. But a recent analysis pooling together results of randomized clinical trials testing hydroxychloroquine's use in early Covid-19 infection should substantially raise the volume.

The hydroxychloroquine saga cannot be fully appreciated without first considering the unusual circumstances under which it arose. While the medical profession has always sustained debate over which treatments are best, the tenor of the hydroxychloroquine controversy is unique. Physicians who have advocated for its effectiveness have remained steadfast in their support of the medication, despite unsupportive clinical trials enrolling hospitalized patients, social media blackouts of their opinions, and a chorus of politicians and health officials telling them—and the country—that they're not only wrong but reckless.

While physicians who hold marginalized or unpopular positions about treatments are often considered by peers to be motivated by profit or other self-serving interests, these physicians were unnoteworthy in that regard, and would largely have been considered "mainstream" prior to the pandemic. Their clinical experiences were dismissed as anecdotal, but consistently achieving patient outcomes that were markedly better than those reported around the country fueled their confidence and tenacity. The nation and the world may now benefit from their steadfastness.

The key data come from randomized trials testing hydroxychloroquine's effectiveness when used to prevent or treat Covid-19 infection in the early stages of disease, while patients are still home and not hospitalized with severe pneumonia. Because they minimize bias, well-performed randomized trials yield weighty clinical evidence. And unlike many of the clinical trials enrolling hospitalized patients, the hydroxychloroquine doses used in outpatient studies have been lower and not in the toxic range.

These lower doses are more aligned with the reputation for safety that hydroxychloroquine has accrued over decades of use in patients with lupus or needing malaria prophylaxis. Studies generally used a dose ranging from 400 mg one day per week for prevention to 600 mg daily for up to one week for treatment, safe for most older adults with comorbidities. Additionally, early treatment is consistent with what we know about the benefits of earlier antiviral therapy for other viral infections, such as oseltamivir (Tamiflu) in influenza, acyclovir in herpes encephalitis, zanamivir for influenza prophylaxis, and HIV antiviral therapy for pre-exposure or post-exposure prophylaxis.

Five of these outpatient randomized trials were published in time to be included in a new analysis, and each reported a benefit for prevention of death, hospitalization or Covid-19 infection that favored hydroxychloroquine use, although no individual study found this benefit to be statistically significant. We used a popular method in health sciences called meta-analysis to pool the results of these randomized trials for the purpose of obtaining a more statistically definitive result. We prioritized analyzing the most meaningful clinical outcomes—death and hospitalization—and analyzed Covid-19 infection rates when these were unavailable.

Our meta-analysis shows that the statistically insignificant results from each of the randomized Covid-19 trials of outpatient hydroxychloroquine translates into a statistically significant 24% risk reduction. In other words, it is evidence from randomized trials that hydroxychloroquine reduces the risk of death, hospitalization or infection from Covid-19 when used for prevention or early treatment.

Even before this meta-analysis, benefits averaging around a 50% risk reduction had already been reported by several non-randomized studies using standard statistical methods to compare health outcomes among people with Covid-19 treated with hydroxychloroquine versus usual care. A site tracking hydroxychloroquine research lists them, which most readers will be surprised to see is replete with outpatient studies reporting reductions in hospitalization and death.

President Trump's recent brush with Covid-19—and the sharp contrast between his treatment and the quarantine-and-wait guidance provided to regular Americans—illustrates how valuable early outpatient therapy could be for millions of vulnerable adults in this country and around the world. Hydroxychloroquine may also play a role in reducing the risk faced by adults who are unwilling or unable to receive a Covid-19 vaccine. The societal benefits of reducing fear due to availability of effective home treatment would be almost immeasurable.

The randomized trials of early outpatient use of hydroxychloroquine, in combination with results from nonrandomized studies, provide very strong evidence of hydroxychloroquine's benefit in the prevention and treatment of Covid-19. While this inexpensive and old medication may not arouse the same intrigue—or avarice—as experimental antibodies or novel antiviral agents, its outpatient use is likely to prevent avoidable deaths. People in the United States and around the world should have access to it, and physicians should feel empowered to prescribe hydroxychloroquine to their vulnerable patients.

Too Much Caution Is Killing Covid Patients[*]
Wall Street Journal, November 24, 2020

Doctors should follow the evidence for promising therapies. Instead they demand certainty.

---

[*] https://www.wsj.com/articles/too-much-caution-is-killing-covid-patients-11606238928.

Fear and panic are central impediments to competent decision-making during a crisis. As Covid-19 cases and hospitalizations rise around the country, creating an atmosphere of crisis, political leaders are reaching for last spring's lockdown playbooks. Their grave tone conveys an air of inevitability, as if politicians have no choice but again to restrict civil liberties, limit social gatherings, and cripple businesses that survived the initial lockdowns. But there's a better way: following the evidence for early treatment of Covid-19.

The health system would be less burdened if more patients were treated before they require hospitalization, and there are promising therapeutic options that patients can administer themselves at home. This was the subject of a Nov. 19 hearing before the Senate Homeland Security and Governmental Affairs Committee.

Testimony from the hearing underscored an important issue: Too many doctors have interpreted the term "evidence-based medicine" to mean that the evidence for a treatment must be certain and definitive before it can be given to patients. Because accusing a physician of not being "evidence based" can be a career-damaging allegation, fear of straying from the pack has prevailed, favoring inertia and inaction amid uncertainty about Covid-19 treatments.

For diseases with established treatment options, holding out for certainty may be prudent. But when options are limited and there are safe treatments with evidence for effectiveness, holding out for certainty can be catastrophic. Requiring a high degree of certainty during a crisis may elevate the augustness of medical organizations and appease the sensibilities of medical professionals, but it does nothing for patients who need help.

The penchant for certainty is visible in the frequently updated treatment guidelines for Covid-19 from the National Institutes of Health. These guidelines were developed by scientists around the country, but because of a mentality that is biased toward virtually irrefutable evidence, no distinction is made for treatments with evidence for effectiveness that falls below the mark of certainty. This framework almost certainly has contributed to many avoidable deaths during this pandemic.

Take the antidepressant fluvoxamine. A high-quality, randomized clinical trial of 152 patients published in the Journal of the American Medical Association found that zero patients treated with fluvoxamine within seven days of the onset of symptoms experienced clinical deterioration compared with 8% of patients receiving a placebo.

Another randomized trial of 200 health-care workers and other adults at high risk of exposure found that 2% of those treated with the antiparasitic ivermectin developed Covid-19 compared with 10% of patients in a control group. A meta-analysis of five randomized clinical trials showed that early use of hydroxychloroquine reduced infection, hospitalization and death by 24%. All of these findings were statistically significant. These medications have been used for decades and have safety profiles comparable to other commonly prescribed medications. This includes hydroxychloroquine, a medication routinely prescribed to pregnant women and breast-feeding mothers.

Uncertainty may remain, but all three medications have demonstrated at least a reasonable likelihood of success when used in early Covid-19 illness or for prevention. Other promising agents include the plant-based compound quercetin—which is being studied in a clinical trial and was used by Sen. Ron Johnson, chairman of the Homeland Security Committee, after his Covid-19 diagnosis in October—and the congestion medication bromhexine, which reduced death rates among hospitalized patients in a randomized study published by BioImpacts.

The evidence for early use of ivermectin and hydroxychloroquine is also supported by studies that weren't randomized, such as a well-designed study published in Travel Medicine and Infectious Disease, along with a study of patients with more advanced disease published in Chest, the journal of the American College of Chest Physicians.

While some health officials dismiss nonrandomized studies, the Cochrane organization, an international leader in evidence-based medicine, published a review of several hundred studies showing that randomized clinical trials and nonrandomized studies of treatments generally yield similar findings. Modern epidemiologic and statistical methods can usually overcome biases inherent in nonrandomized study designs.

The most auspicious path forward is for local and state governments, research institutions, community clinics and Covid-19 testing sites to provide patients with access to promising outpatient treatments while collecting data about health outcomes. With almost 200,000 new Covid-19 cases daily in the U. S., uncertainty about effectiveness could be resolved within a few weeks. Until then, it is up to patients to demand outpatient treatment. Political leaders have largely been silent, and most physicians have been telling Covid-19 patients to quarantine and hope for the best rather than prescribing early treatment.

As California Gov. Gavin Newsom recently demonstrated with his festive dinner party at a Napa Valley restaurant, asking human beings not to socialize is neither realistic nor healthy. Attempting to shame them into cooperating runs counter to fundamental tenets of public health. And while masks may be effective in crowded or poorly ventilated indoor settings, the recent randomized trial of mask use in Denmark—along with Covid-19 case trends in California, New York and other states that have had mask mandates in place for months—should disabuse anyone of the illusion that mask mandates will quell the crisis.

Treating high-risk patients with Covid-19 at home using safe medications is the most promising public-health strategy for preventing hospital overcrowding and death. These treatments are widely available and can be combined with other measures. What Americans need in this crisis is clear-eyed policy inspired by imagination and a genuine desire to protect the vulnerable—rather than fueled by fear or partisan political agendas.

CHAPTER 11

COVID-19 Vaccines: Ideology versus Science

Clear thinking is never more critical than during a crisis. Ironically, the pressures of a crisis also make us particularly vulnerable to abandoning clear thinking and instead reaching for "comfort" strategies, such as mental shortcuts and fantastical beliefs.

Clear thinking is characterized by leaders speaking plainly about the circumstances of a crisis, acknowledging uncertainty and limitations, and proposing sensible plans that are presented as works in progress possibly needing modification in the future. Conversely, a lack of clarity and rational thought is always revealed by confused communication, denial of uncertainty and limitations, and demands for strict adherence to "the plan"—though that plan may not be supported by current facts or historical lessons.

When pharmaceutical companies first developed COVID-19 vaccines and announced their efficacy results in November 2020, the public health community had the option of taking the path of clear thinking. Specifically, this would have meant acknowledging the fact that there were many unknowns about safety, deploying a vaccine dissemination strategy that respected personal choice, and remaining open to the possibility that efficacy reports from drug manufacturers might not align with real-world data.

I had no expectation this would happen, however, given the abysmal track record of most leaders during the pandemic. Not only had they made countless poor decisions and embraced senseless—and often harmful—public policy, but there seemed to be no self-awareness about these failures or how they might do better in the future.

To understand how and why the public health community fell short, and how we can avoid these mistakes in the future, I have divided this chapter into six sections. The first section sets the stage for why clear thinking in the face of COVID-19 vaccines was bound to be a challenge. I discuss the elephant in the room, which is the indoctrination surrounding vaccines that occurs in medical education. With this background, the second section discusses early scientific considerations in the lead-up to COVID-19 vaccine availability that were most relevant to health policy, and the third section analyzes the "get everyone vaccinated" strategy that became a viral sensation among public health leaders.

In the fourth section, I describe a simple framework for considering COVID-19 vaccine safety. In the fifth section, I discuss reactions I received at UCLA after discussing COVID-19 vaccine safety publicly. And in the final section, I discuss why the safety of COVID-19 vaccines will likely be a defining aspect of public health's legacy in relation to this pandemic.

Medical School Vaccine Indoctrination

The public health community will have to disentangle itself from its indoctrinated beliefs about vaccines if it ever hopes to make unbiased and clearheaded policy recommendations during health crises. This is not a statement "for" or "against" vaccines, nor is that at all relevant to the concept of indoctrination. This is a statement about how education is provided, how beliefs are acquired, and how these things shape our interpretation of data and outlook about policy.

The education that physicians receive about vaccines during medical school is unlike the education we receive about any other therapy. With most therapies, there is usually discussion about risks and benefits, technical aspects of use such as dosing and frequency, and alternative therapeutic agents. This information is normally provided without celebration or critique and is presented in a matter-of-fact way. For example, statins, which are by far the most effective and affordable drugs for preventing cardiovascular disease in high-risk patients, are presented in this manner—without positive or negative bias.

With vaccines, however, while there is discussion about risks and benefits and dosing, the discussion is enshrouded in a belief system about how "good" vaccines are and how individuals who criticize them have inherently invalid positions. Vaccines are literally praised rather than discussed in an even-handed manner that nurtures the student's ability to reach his or her own conclusions. In other words, the education in this area takes on the quality of indoctrination. Based on my experience, our colleagues in schools of public health undergo similar indoctrination.

I myself was a disciple of this doctrine, and it took the COVID-19 pandemic and directly witnessing gross misrepresentations of scientific findings and dismissal of valid COVID-19 vaccine safety concerns to awaken me. This led me to reexamine my own beliefs and how I came to have them.

This indoctrination of doctors to treat vaccines as sacrosanct is, of course, an enormous boon to pharmaceutical companies. To manufacture and profit from a product that, by default, is reflexively protected by medical doctors—arguably the most respected of all professions—and receives the benefit of the doubt when questions of safety arise is an extraordinary arrangement. Yet, despite the fact that most physicians are unfamiliar with the primary scientific studies that inform safety and effectiveness of different vaccines, we readily pledge our loyalty.

For a historical perspective on the issue and more contextual information about the politics, I refer readers to Robert F. Kennedy Jr.'s book *The Real Anthony Fauci*. However one feels about the subject matter, the facts he provides are well-referenced.

For example, RFK Jr. mentions a statement in the Federal Register Vol. 49, No.107, June 1, 1984, that left me in disbelief. The Federal Register is a record of United States government's agency rules and public notices. I tracked down the 1984 version (it is available online at a government website) to confirm RFK Jr.'s reference and was shocked when I read the passage myself.

In reference to the oral polio vaccine, the Federal Register states: "However, although the continued availability of the vaccine may not be in immediate jeopardy, any possible doubts, whether or not well founded, about the safety of the vaccine cannot be allowed to exist in view of the need to assure that the vaccine will continue to be used to the maximum extent consistent with the nation's public health objectives."

The FDA, which authored this section of the Federal Register, does present a "justification" for their remarkable endorsement of dishonesty. After all, there are often at least two sides to any controversial issue. But the frank admission that "well founded" doubts should not be "allowed to exist" is obviously extraordinary and would inspire a lively debate about government ethics.

Another area that was not covered in medical school but is of absolute importance if a leader seeks to make the wisest decisions possible is a field that studies "nonspecific effects" of vaccines. This basically means "unanticipated" effects that are unplanned and unrelated to the protection a vaccine confers to a disease. Considering the near-infinite complexities of the human body and particularly our immune systems, it should not be surprising that cells interact in unanticipated and unpredictable ways.

One particular area of inquiry in "nonspecific effects" is the evaluation of a vaccine's effects on mortality. An emblematic article in this area is a 2020 review published in *The Lancet Infectious Diseases* by Dr. Christine Stabell Benn, a professor at the University of Southern Denmark. The scientific question being posed was simple: What are the effects of different vaccines on a person's overall survival?

For example, prior studies showed that a diphtheria-tetanus-pertussis (DTP) vaccine was associated with increased mortality in girls, but not in boys, and a high-tier measles vaccine was withdrawn after it was associated with a doubling in mortality risk in girls, but not in boys. Some vaccines seemed to affect overall mortality differently depending on the order in which they were given.

More recently, a malaria vaccine was associated with higher all-cause mortality in girls. All of these vaccines protected against the diseases for which they were designed, but the physiological responses they elicited led to detrimental effects on other diseases or conditions, thereby increasing mortality. The news was not all bad: for example, the Bacille Calmette-Guérin (BCG) vaccine for tuberculosis was found to *reduce* childhood mortality for reasons unrelated to tuberculosis. However, the point is that vaccines have nonspecific effects that can only be known after they are in use.

Each of these discoveries exemplifies an issue that is relevant to vaccine safety, relevant to public health policy and leadership, and relevant to how to develop a thoughtful approach to COVID-19 vaccine policymaking. But our current culture of indoctrination prevents people from asking questions that should be asked.

COVID-19 Vaccine Data Debut

There were two major factors that influenced the potential direction of health policy around the time Pfizer and Moderna released their vaccine trial results in November 2020. The first factor was the substantial gap between anticipated and reported efficacy. The second factor was the dearth of information about the vaccines' effects on preventing serious COVID-19 illness.

A third factor, which was so ahead of its time as to not be influential, was an early and concrete safety concern. In a comment sent to the FDA on December 8, 2020, Dr. J. Patrick Whelan of UCLA presciently warned about an increased risk of myocarditis or other organ injury from the vaccines. But wider recognition of this would have to wait.

Returning to the first major factor: earlier in the pandemic, the FDA had announced that any COVID-19 vaccine would have to be at least 50 percent effective in preventing disease to receive authorization. But Pfizer was reporting an effectiveness rate that exceeded 95 percent, and Moderna was soon to follow. This caught many scientists by surprise. Because of the large gap between expectations and reported findings, there was sure to be some shake-up in how researchers and the public health community viewed the vaccines. Unfortunately, this shake-up made things worse and not better because it ultimately fueled the "shot into every arm" obsession.

The early evidence portending this outcome was visible in how health officials sincerely described the vaccines as the first sign of "hope" during the pandemic, and in how intently every mile of the journey that FedEx trucks took from distribution centers to vaccination sites was followed. It was as if the vaccines were being worshipped—a clear indicator that magical thinking would continue and Americans would continue to suffer under pandemic crusaders.

In counterbalance, the second major factor was a concern about the adequacy of the COVID-19 vaccine trials, as vocalized by a sizable portion of the scientific community. Their concerns represented lingering vestiges of clear thinking, although they would soon be overtaken by the "vaccinate everyone" crowd. The general tenor of this group was that the number of "events" (COVID-19 cases or incidences of COVID-19 illness) was too small to provide us with meaningful information about how clinically useful the vaccines were.

A good example of the concerns raised by this group was published in the *New York Times* on Sept. 22, 2020. Written by Dr. Peter Doshi, a professor at the University of Maryland School of Pharmacy and senior editor at *The BMJ*, and Dr. Eric Topol, a cardiologist and founder of the Scripps Research Translational Institute in San Diego, the article argued that the COVID-19 vaccine clinical trials wouldn't answer the question of whether the vaccines reduced the risk of serious illness from COVID-19. This was because the clinical trials generally required only evidence of mild symptoms and a positive COVID-19 test for a participant to be considered a "case." Because mild cases were, on average, more than ten times as frequent as cases requiring hospitalization, clinical trials could have satisfied FDA's requirements for authorization while not showing any improvements in preventing hospitalization or death.

As an aside, Peter, who is a friend of mine, has remained inquisitive in his research on the data supporting much of COVID-19 pandemic policymaking, whereas Eric has largely abandoned critical appraisal of any evidence that casts the vaccines in a negative light.

Fortunately, later data would show that the COVID-19 vaccines were generally effective at reducing the risk of severe COVID-19 illness, but it was unfortunate that such an important issue fell to the wayside in pursuit of universal vaccination. Moreover, the "get everyone vaccinated" obsession was just another example of how little mental clarity public health leaders possessed at this stage of the pandemic.

"A Shot Into Every Arm"

Soon after vaccine efficacy data were available, an obsessive campaign to "vaccinate everyone" became an almost uniform refrain from public health officials in the United States. This was unfortunate, since it lacked the quality of mindful leadership that allows one to see things for what they *are* rather than what we wish they were. But mindful leadership and indoctrination are completely incompatible, and the latter was well-seated in the minds of most health officials.

It was clear from how the pandemic had evolved that there were basically two types of Americans that public health officials should have been considering in their development of vaccine policy. The first type were Americans who could literally not feel "safe" coming out of their houses or being around other people without first receiving a vaccine. (Ironically, we would later learn that many of these people still would not feel safe afterward.) The second type were Americans who had grown weary of pandemic restrictions and just wanted to get on with life.

The people in the first group would fill the long stretches of lines at mass vaccination sites, whereas the people in the second group might show up months later when lines thinned, or they might not show up at all. Moreover, some of the people in this group were deeply opposed to how fear had been weaponized as a public health tool and were consequently opposed to contributing to this environment by receiving a vaccine they did not feel they needed.

Instead of appreciating these differences and incorporating them in pandemic policy, most public health leadership felt that everyone had to receive the vaccine, often stating that this was the only way to "end the pandemic." Not only did this prove to be factually incorrect, as we would soon learn from epidemiological data on infections and reinfections in people receiving COVID-19 vaccines, but it also fed rifts and created substantial antagonism among many people in the second category, who felt their autonomy was being subverted. So the campaign was both scientifically flawed and unwise.

I wrote about the foolishness of this approach in an article that was published in the *Wall Street Journal* on February 4, 2021. As I typed out a draft at my desk in our Los Angeles home, I chose my words carefully, more so than I had ever done in the past. I chose my words so carefully because of my awareness that vaccines hold a special place in the tomes of medical knowledge and that any analysis that does not cast them in an unequivocally positive light is often considered heretical. This is perhaps one of the major hurdles hampering the medical community's ability to be a trustworthy source of guidance during health crises. I describe this in more detail in the next section.

COVID-19 Vaccine Safety

As a rule, in the field of medicine, we always learn more about the safety of therapies over time. The hope, of course, is that this new knowledge does not lead to a reversal of the recommendation for a medication's use in the future. But evolving knowledge about the safety of a therapy is the rule rather than the exception in medical science. And this knowledge should lead a mindful leader to carry a modicum of caution when promoting new therapies.

With COVID-19 vaccines, much of public health leadership seems to have forgotten this lesson. The "shot into every arm" evangelists skipped the exercise of performing rigorous and trustworthy risk-benefit calculations and recommended the vaccines as doggedly for older Americans as they did for children, even though the risk of death from COVID-19 was up to 1,000 times higher in the former group. It made no sense. The pace of efforts to promote adoption was completely mismatched with our knowledge about safety.

The resounding message from the public health community has been that the vaccines are "safe and effective." The leading argument to support this position is that "millions of Americans" had already received a COVID-19 vaccine, with the implication that they must be safe since so many had received a dose. But there were two problems with this argument.

The first problem was that it was obvious to any honest individual that the media and physicians largely and intentionally ignored individuals who reported adverse events after their vaccination, and social media companies explicitly censored this content. Articles that described the death of an individual shortly after COVID-19 vaccination, for example, were tethered to "fact checker" articles that regaled readers with clumsy explanations about how a connection between the two was impossible. The amount of scientific dishonesty was unlike anything I had witnessed in my scientific career. So the fact that millions had received the vaccine was no bellwether of safety, given the strong public bias to suppress concerns about adverse events.

The second problem with the argument was that there was another vaccine that over 100 million Americans received each year but that had elicited nowhere near the same degree of concerns about safety. This was the seasonal influenza vaccine. With very few exceptions, the most common complaint people had after influenza vaccination was that "it gave me the flu." Based on my years of experience as a physician, reports of adverse events after COVID 19 vaccination were far more prevalent, by orders of magnitude, and far more severe.

With this in mind, I wrote an article in the *Wall Street Journal* published on April 19, 2021, that highlighted the fact that risk-benefit balance of the vaccines in low-risk populations like children was truly unknown. Dr. Harvey Risch and I followed this up with an article about vaccine-associated adverse events in the *Wall Street Journal* on June 22, 2021.

Both of these articles were examples of clear thinking during a crisis: we approached the issue with honesty and integrity, rather than by making overstatements about things that were uncertain or feverishly projecting our desires on the wills of others (in contrast to the public health crowd determined to "end the pandemic," whatever the price). In addition, I wrote an unpublished article about the short-sightedness and scientific arrogance inherent in a mass vaccination campaign with a new vaccine technology.

An additional layer of injustice in COVID-19 vaccine safety politics is how adverse event complaints from the general public are frequently dismissed by physicians, but complaints about adverse events made by individuals in the scientific community are taken more seriously. I have received countless reports of the former from patients, friends, and even strangers across the country. It's heartbreaking.

But when someone like Dr. Gregory Poland, the director of Mayo Clinic's Vaccine Research Group, developed severe tinnitus within about ninety minutes of receiving his second dose of an mRNA COVID-19 vaccine, the possibility of a linkage received more attention.

"We really do need more research in this area," he said in a Healio interview. And in a MedPage Today interview, he shared, "What has been heartbreaking about this, as a seasoned physician, are the emails I get from people that, this has affected their life so badly, they have told me they are going to take their own life."

Stories like this deeply sadden me, both because of how people are suffering and because much of the scientific community believes that defending the "safe and effective" messaging about COVID-19 vaccines is more important than defending truth and honesty. It also happens to be a foolhardy strategy. Eventually, whatever the truth is regarding the safety of these COVID-19 vaccines—particularly the mRNA vaccines—will be known. If doctors have misled people in pursuit of a public health goal, will redemption be easily recovered? Widespread loss of public trust in physicians will be *devastating*. Being honest in the face of uncertainty would have been an infinitely wiser strategy.

Individuals whose response to Dr. Poland's story is to say, "Well, COVID-19 can cause tinnitus too," miss the point. It would be like someone who was a victim of child abuse in the Catholic church being told that other churches have also had cases of child abuse. The point is about honesty and integrity, not about what's happening in your neighbor's house.

Are the risks associated with COVID-19 relevant? Of course. But that leads to a different and distinct question. The question is not whether

COVID-19 is associated with its own risks, but rather whether the benefits outweigh the risks of COVID-19 vaccination.

That question encapsulates both the risks of tinnitus associated with the vaccine and the risk of tinnitus associated with infection, along with the probabilities of these outcomes, along with the balance of other risks and benefits associated with either strategy. That is the correct question to answer. To put it differently, even if the risk of developing tinnitus was 100 percent after COVID-19 infection, receiving a COVID-19 vaccine would be the worse strategy if the chance of infection was nil due to prior immunity (not the case, but I am stating this for the purpose of example) or the absence of community transmission.

Fallout at UCLA

I share the reactions to my articles about vaccine safety and proper consideration of risks and benefits so the reader can gain a fuller sense of the degree of indoctrination that occurs with vaccines in the medical community.

It started with the usual mix of public reactions. Strangers emailed me at my UCLA account to either thank me for my honesty or to share their hopes that I die a painful death from the virus. Many reached out solely to deliver their acrimonious assessment of me as a human being.

One member of UCLA's research community charitably cc'd me on an email to the chancellor with a subject line of "Why does UCLA employ Dr. Ladapo?" He whined that my article would "hurt our efforts to vaccinate the country" and reminded the chancellor that "Stanford has taken public stands when Dr. Scott Atlas did similar things."

Closer to my academic home, a UCLA infectious disease doctor who was an investigator on one of my HIV research studies, and whose kids had attended the same birthday parties as my own children, decided it was time to pursue disownment. "The idea of diverse opinions stops when there are threats (cloaked and otherwise) to human rights or public health," she wrote. "It certainly comes off as a matter of pure self-interest. . . . I regret that I will not agree to being an author on any further publications with you."

Even closer to home, my division chief, Dr. Carol Mangione, told me that the medical school dean would be joining our next one-on-one meeting. Not in the mood for an ambush or tag-team effort to wear me down, I declined to participate and insisted that future communications about anything related to my editorials be in writing. In her defense, I know that Dr. Mangione was in a difficult position and that she had beaten back many attempts by members of the UCLA community to somehow punish me for my writings.

All this time, I was becoming more and more an "outsider" at UCLA, and a bit of an oddity. I was surprised when, while taking care of patients at Ronald Reagan UCLA Medical Center, a medical resident on my team told me that several of his colleagues had asked what it was like working with me. "I told them you are very reasonable, thoughtful, and listen to other people's perspectives," he said. The feedback he shared was met with surprise. I shuddered to think of the stories people were telling themselves about me.

Ultimately, these reactions illustrate the degree of indoctrination that existed in my local medical community about vaccines in general and COVID-19 vaccines in particular, but sadly, they also showed how close-minded this community was. My ideas were far from "radical," and the rationale for them was clearly laid out in the articles I wrote. But it is impossible to have rational debates with an indoctrinated audience if the subject you are debating is perceived to be a threat to their belief system. The whole thing is an unfortunate commentary on medical education in general.

Vaccine Safety as a Defining Aspect of Public Health's COVID-19 Legacy

The legacy of this pandemic for the public health community will be shaped in part by the "final" answers about vaccine safety, specifically with respect to the mRNA vaccines developed by Pfizer and Moderna. The reason is that health officials and medical doctors literally placed all their eggs in one basket, so much so that they supported obnoxious vaccine passports, inhumane firings of nurses and firefighters who declined vaccination, and prolonged infringement of civil liberties with public health mandates and restrictions.

The commitment of the public health community was so absolute that they managed to rouse record levels of distrust, particularly among the large proportion of the country that is politically conservative or Republican. They also inspired distrust in other areas, such as with routine childhood vaccines. I know parents who are now newly demurring on regular childhood vaccines because of the scientific shenanigans they witnessed during the pandemic.

COVID-19 vaccine mandates in particular crossed a special line; based on pure common sense, how can something be mandated when it is not even effective at stopping viral spread? (See an article I wrote in the *Wall Street Journal* on September 16, 2021, for more about this.)

The misrepresentations and moral compromises that have been made by the scientific community in the name of persuading or coercing individuals to take one, two, three, and now four (and counting) COVID-19 vaccines are probably an appropriate climax to what has been an extraordinary series of poor pandemic decisions. The public health community's decisions will define their legacy because they championed profoundly disruptive—and ultimately ineffective—policies. Already, data that show a worsening of educational achievement gaps are emerging as a major—albeit underreported—issue. If rigorous data analyses show definitively that benefits did not outweigh risks for the major populations for which COVID-19 vaccines were recommended, public health—and medicine as we know it—will struggle to recover. In that sense, this chapter remains unfinished . . . at least for now.

The Universal Vaccination' Chimera*
Wall Street Journal, February 4, 2021

Tools for stopping variants are limited and, like masks and distancing, vaccines are not a panacea.

---

* https://www.wsj.com/articles/the-universal-vaccination-chimera-11612466130.

Each stage of the American Covid-19 pandemic has been marked by a singular public-health message that crowded out all other perspectives. From early calls to "crush the curve" with shutdowns and pleas to stay at home, then to claims that face masks would end the pandemic, these messaging strategies have sowed unrealistic expectations and delayed public acceptance of reality. The most recent message is "universal vaccination," an aspiration whose unattainability may further delay the country's return to social and economic normalcy.

How did we arrive at this point in the pandemic? The media's campaign to stoke fear about collapsing health systems, along with their portrayal of severe illness as the inevitable consequence of infection—despite a thousandfold difference in risk between old and young—contributed to an atmosphere of distrust. Animosity toward Donald Trump —justified or not—fueled this campaign. Health officials abetted the discord by abandoning longstanding public-health tenets that emphasize harm reduction and a non-judgmental outlook. Instead, these experts promoted mandates for the healthy and public shaming of people who strayed from guidelines.

Now the fear and distrust have made a substantial proportion of the U.S. population unreceptive to a vaccine. While vaccine receptiveness might be expected to vary based on a person's risk of illness, a January Gallup survey showed that a stronger predictor is political preference. More than 80% of Democrats are willing to be vaccinated, but only about 45% of Republicans are.

The long vaccination lines seen on television will eventually thin as Americans most worried about contracting Covid-19 receive their shots. Many of the estimated 100 million Americans who aren't interested in vaccination are unlikely to change their decision voluntarily.

What also isn't serving vaccination efforts: the lack of transparent communication from public-health officials that meets people where they are and sincerely acknowledges the concerns of millions who view Covid-19 vaccines with suspicion. Concerns have been dismissed or derided as "misinformation." It's true that serious adverse effects appear to be uncommon, according to Centers for Disease Control and Prevention reports. But responding to these worries by insisting more loudly that the vaccines are safe isn't an effective strategy. A wiser strategy is to address these concerns with data about what is known, and honesty and humility about areas of uncertainty—such as vaccination in pregnant women.

The expert insistence that Covid-19 vaccination is a social responsibility, that getting vaccinated is "doing your part," is a political philosophy and not a self-evident truth. The natural instinct driving most health behavior—much like wearing a mask last spring before mandates—is self-preservation. Altruism is a virtue and makes everyone better off, but it is foolish to rely on it as a public-health strategy. Moreover, while scientists argue that widespread vaccination will prevent variants from taking hold, lessons from the past year should make it abundantly clear that our ability to stop the spread of variants is extraordinarily limited.

The possibility of Covid-19 vaccine mandates in schools deserves special attention. There are almost no data on the potential benefits or harms of Covid-19 vaccination in children, and no crystal ball to predict disease epidemiology in a future that will likely include high vaccination rates among teachers and vulnerable family members. Yet at least one school district—Los Angeles Unified, the nation's second largest—has announced it intends to require the vaccine for students.

Even amid assurances from scientists, many parents will remain skeptical about vaccinating their children. This is reasonable, considering that a study in the leading journal Nature estimated the Covid-19 survival rate to be approximately 99.995% in children and teens. By contrast, measles leads to hospitalization in about 1 in 5 unvaccinated persons, according to the CDC. What school officials are asking these parents to do is give up their parental intuition and give way to "expert opinion." These battles will be tremendous, and wiser leadership would avoid them by considering other options, such as symptom monitoring or periodic testing.

A sensible and sustainable approach to vaccine policy would focus access on two populations: Americans who are at high risk of severe disease, and Americans who may be at lower risk but feel they can't live and work safely without vaccination. This will free up resources and attention for tackling other challenges, such as attrition among people who need a second vaccine dose, and virus variants that may blunt vaccine protection. Some 90% of deaths from Covid-19 are among those over 55; the death rate would be expected to plummet if the older and vulnerable were protected effectively.

Other forces pushing mortality lower: The CDC estimates that approximately 83 million Americans contracted Covid-19 through December. Reinfection risk is low for at least six to nine months following infection. There is also growing scientific evidence for outpatient therapies such as ivermectin, colchicine, fluvoxamine and the politically charged hydroxychloroquine, as well as better hospital practices.

A sharp decline in mortality will give rational thinking a bigger stage, allowing schools to reopen and social and economic activities to resume. It will also liberate American society from the fear-fueled decision-making that has dominated the pandemic response.

An American Epidemic of 'Covid Mania'*
Wall Street Journal, April 19, 2021

The problem isn't only the overreaction to the virus but the diminution of every other problem.

What are the lessons of Covid-19? It depends who you ask. Some believe politicization of the pandemic response cost lives. Others believe a stronger U.S. public-health system would have reduced

---

* https://www.wsj.com/articles/an-american-epidemic-of-covid-mania-11618871457.

Covid-19 deaths significantly. Still others say lockdowns should have been longer and more stringent, or that they were ineffective. But one lesson that should transcend ideological differences: Don't put one illness above all other problems in society, a condition known as "Covid mania."

The novel coronavirus has caused suffering and heartbreak, particularly for older adults and their loved ones. But it also has a low mortality rate among most people and especially the young—estimated at 0.01% for people under 40—and therefore never posed a serious threat to social and economic institutions. Compassion and realism need not be enemies. But Covid mania crowded out reasoned and wise policy making.

Americans groaned when leaders first called for "two weeks to slow the spread" in March 2020. Months later, many of these same Americans hardly blinked when leaders declared that lockdowns should continue indefinitely. For months Covid had been elevated above all other problems in society. Over time new rules were written and new norms accepted.

Liberty has played a special role in U.S. history, fueling advances from independence to emancipation to the fight for equal rights for women and racial minorities. Unfortunately, Covid mania led many policy makers to treat liberty as a nuisance rather than a core American principle.

Covid mania has also wreaked havoc on science and its influence on policy. While scientists' passion for discovery and improving health has fueled research on the novel coronavirus, Covid mania has interpreted scientific advancements through an increasingly narrow frame. There has only been one question: How can scientific findings be deployed to reduce Covid-19 spread? It hasn't mattered how impractical these measures may be. Discoveries that might have helped save lives, such as better outpatient therapies, were ignored because they didn't fit the desired policy outcome.

A prime example is mask research. However one feels about wearing masks, look at the evidence from California. Despite a mask mandate imposed last April and steady, high rates of compliance, California experienced a surge in Covid-19 cases over the winter.

Mandating masks may help in some settings, but masks are not the panacea officials have presented them as. In September, then-Centers for Disease Control and Prevention director Robert Redfield declared that "this face mask is more guaranteed to protect me against Covid than when I take a Covid vaccine."

The statement was remarkable because he made it before seeing vaccine trial data. Those data and data from people who have recovered from Covid clearly demonstrate that this statement is false. Immunity is far more effective than whatever efficacy masks may offer.

Covid mania is also creating new conflicts over vaccine mandates. The same people who assured the public that a few weeks of lockdown would control the pandemic now argue that vaccinating children, for whom no vaccine has yet been approved, is essential to end the pandemic. Children account for less than 0.1% of Covid deaths in the U.S. Is enough known about vaccines to conclude that their benefits outweigh potential risks to children?

"Yes" is the answer of a salesman, not a scientist. Mandating a vaccine for children without knowing whether the benefits outweigh the risks is unethical. People who insist we should press on anyway, because variants will prolong the pandemic, should be reminded that a large reservoir of unvaccinated people in the U.S.—and in the world—will always exist. We cannot outrun the variants.

The good news is that recent state legislative efforts in Utah, Tennessee and Ohio to ban vaccine passports may burst the Covid mania bubble. If passports are banned, then risks from Covid must be assessed in the same way other risks—such as playing a sport or starting a new medication—are considered. In many places throughout the country, zero has become the only tolerable risk level. Why else are people who have been vaccinated or recovered from Covid still asked to wear masks? Reasonable policies cannot sprout from unreasonable levels of risk tolerance.

The pandemic has been devastating for many Americans, but policies grounded in Covid mania have compounded the harm and delayed a return to normal life. The challenges ahead require rational decision making that considers costs and benefits and keeps sight of the countless things in life that matter.

Are Covid Vaccines Riskier Than Advertised?[*]
Wall Street Journal, June 22, 2021

There are concerning trends on blood clots and low platelets, not that the authorities will tell you.

One remarkable aspect of the Covid-19 pandemic has been how often unpopular scientific ideas, from the lab-leak theory to the efficacy of masks, were initially dismissed, even ridiculed, only to resurface later in mainstream thinking. Differences of opinion have sometimes been rooted in disagreement over the underlying science. But the more common motivation has been political.

Another reversal in thinking may be imminent. Some scientists have raised concerns that the safety risks of Covid-19 vaccines have been underestimated. But the politics of vaccination has relegated their concerns to the outskirts of scientific thinking—for now.

Historically, the safety of medications—including vaccines—is often not fully understood until they are deployed in large populations. Examples include rofecoxib (Vioxx), a pain reliever that increased the risk of heart attack and stroke; antidepressants that appeared to increase suicide attempts among young adults; and an influenza vaccine used in the 2009-10 swine flu epidemic that was suspected of causing febrile convulsions and narcolepsy in children. Evidence from the real world is valuable, as clinical trials often enroll patients who aren't representative of the general population.

---

[*] https://www.wsj.com/articles/are-covid-vaccines-riskier-than-advertised-11624381749.

We learn more about drug safety from real-world evidence and can adjust clinical recommendations to balance risk and benefits.

The Vaccine Adverse Event Reporting System, or Vaers, which is administered by the Centers for Disease Control and Prevention and the Food and Drug Administration, is a database that allows Americans to document adverse events that happen after receiving a vaccine. The FDA and CDC state that the database isn't designed to determine whether the events were caused by a vaccine. This is true. But the data can nonetheless be evaluated, accounting for its strengths and weaknesses, and that is what the CDC and FDA say they do.

The Vaers data for Covid-19 vaccines show an interesting pattern. Among the 310 million Covid-19 vaccines given, several adverse events are reported at high rates in the days immediately after vaccination, and then fall precipitously afterward. Some of these adverse events might have occurred anyway. The pattern may be partly attributable to the tendency to report more events that happen soon after vaccination.

The database can't say what would have happened in the absence of vaccination. Nonetheless, the large clustering of certain adverse events immediately after vaccination is concerning, and the silence around these potential signals of harm reflects the politics surrounding Covid-19 vaccines. Stigmatizing such concerns is bad for scientific integrity and could harm patients.

Four serious adverse events follow this arc, according to data taken directly from Vaers: low platelets (thrombocytopenia); non-infectious myocarditis, or heart inflammation, especially for those under 30; deep-vein thrombosis; and death. Vaers records 321 cases of myocarditis within five days of receiving a vaccination, falling to almost zero by 10 days. Prior research has shown that only a fraction of adverse events are reported, so the true number of cases is almost certainly higher. This tendency of underreporting is consistent with our clinical experience.

Analyses to confirm or dismiss these findings should be per-formed using large data sets of health-insurance companies and healthcare organizations. The CDC and FDA are surely aware of these data patterns, yet neither agency has acknowledged the trend.

The implication is that the risks of a Covid-19 vaccine may outweigh the benefits for certain low-risk populations, such as children, young adults and people who have recovered from Covid-19. This is especially true in regions with low levels of community spread, since the likelihood of illness depends on exposure risk.

And while you would never know it from listening to public-health officials, not a single published study has demonstrated that patients with a prior infection benefit from Covid-19 vaccination. That this isn't readily acknowledged by the CDC or Anthony Fauci is an indication of how deeply entangled pandemic politics is in science.

There are, however, signs of life for scientific honesty. In May, the Norwegian Medicines Agency reviewed case files for the first 100 reported deaths of nursing-home residents who received the Pfizer vaccine. The agency concluded that the vaccine "likely" contributed to the deaths of 10 of these residents through side effects such as fever and diarrhea, and "possibly" contributed to the deaths of an additional 26. But this type of honesty is rare. And it is rare for any vaccine to be linked to deaths, so this unusual development for mRNA vaccines merits further investigation.

The battle to recover scientific honesty will be an uphill one in the U.S. Anti-Trump politics in the spring of 2020 mushroomed into social-media censorship. News reporting often lacked intellectual curiosity about the appropriateness of public-health guidelines—or why a vocal minority of scientists strongly disagreed with prevailing opinions. Scientists have advocated for or against Covid-19 therapies while having financial relationships with product manufacturers and their foundation benefactors.

Public-health authorities are making a mistake and risking the public's trust by not being forthcoming about the possibility of harm from certain vaccine side effects. There will be lasting consequences from mingling political partisanship and science during the management of a public-health crisis.

Have We Learned All There Is to Know About the Safety of COVID-19 Vaccines?
Unpublished, August 5, 2021

Who really believes that we have learned all there is to know about the safety of COVID-19 vaccines after eight months of use in the US population? Few physicians with training in epidemiology would answer in the affirmative. And if a full picture of their safety cannot be known in eight months, how can it be sensible to mandate the vaccines now? The future identification of a meaningful safety risk could have profound ramifications for organizations and governments who follow the path of early mandates. The vaccines represent a new technology, and mandating them now is an enormous gamble.

As we enter this new juncture in the COVID-19 pandemic, it is important to remember how critical missteps over the past 18 months were born out of dogma that outpaced scientific evidence. From lockdowns that now appear to have increased excess deaths according to a recent study from the National Bureau of Economic Research, to prolonged school closures that disproportionately harmed the children of racial/ethnic minorities and damaged the emotional health of countless others, to a yearlong campaign promoting face-mask wearing without acknowledging the conflicting evidence for their use and near uselessness outdoors, unbiased assessments of data have been in short supply. COVID-19 vaccine mandates may become another notch in this belt of failures.

The common argument supporting mandates—and accelerated FDA approval—is that millions of doses of Pfizer and Moderna vaccines have been administered in the United States and peer reviewed studies have not identified major safety signals. Therefore, the vaccines are safe, and, in light of efficacy data, mandates are justified. There are two problems with this argument, and they can be examined without elevating or impugning the safety of the vaccines.

The first problem, which should be apparent to anyone paying attention over this past year and a half, is that data informing decisions have frequently been politicized. This makes it hard to trust—and even harder to determine the truth.

One example of this is how the CDC performed their risk-benefit analysis of COVID-19 vaccination in adolescents and young adults, which concluded that benefits outweighed risk. In what was a brazen analytic decision, the CDC used reports of myocarditis in the Vaccine Adverse Event Reporting System (VAERS) system to estimate incidence, rather than the actual incidence. Not only does VAERS underestimate the incidence of adverse events, but higher quality data from Israel demonstrated an incidence of myocarditis that was five times higher than the CDC's estimate. This decision may have altered the recommendation for vaccination in healthy adolescent boys. In the context of COVID-19, we are not living in a period where honesty and transparency are embraced.

A second example is the fact that, since the Norwegian Medicines Agency reported in May 2021 that Pfizer's COVID-19 vaccine likely contributed to 10 out of the first 100 deaths of vaccinated nursing-home residents, the CDC does not appear to have performed a comparable investigation in the United States. The fact that a governmental agency found a link between vaccination and death is already extraordinary, but the absence of a public CDC response speaks to serious problems with data and transparency.

A third example is the limited public transparency about the CDC's vaccine-safety monitoring system, which includes the Vaccine Safety Datalink (VSD) and other clinical data systems. Louder calls for mandates and accelerated FDA approval should clearly be coupled with greater public disclosure of safety data if integrity and honesty are priorities. The safety reports available to the public and from Advisory Committee on Immunization Practices meetings have been narrowly focused.

The second problem with the argument for mandates is that the safety of many medications—including vaccines—is only fully appreciated over time. Two vaccine-related examples particularly stand out, as described recently in *The Lancet*.

The first example is the bacillus Calmette–Guérin (BCG) vaccine. While the vaccine was developed to protect against tuberculosis, researchers found many years later that children who received certain strains of the live vaccine experienced reductions in overall mortality for reasons unrelated to tuberculosis. This serendipitous finding could not have been known without the benefit of time.

On the other end of the spectrum is the example of the Diphtheria-tetanus-pertussis (DTP) vaccine. Years after its deployment, researchers found that it increased overall mortality, particularly in girls, despite providing protection against the pathogens it targeted. The mechanisms are not fully understood, but what is clearly true is there is much we do not know, and are only likely to discover, over time.

Some policy analysts have supported mandates due to fears about business or organizational liability risk in the short term from exposing employees, patrons, or students to COVID-19. However, other reasonable methods to limit spread exist, including the use of personal protective equipment and routine testing. Importantly, because vaccines and recovering from natural infection have both been shown to reduce the risk of serious COVID illness, much of the policy anguish over masks, public health restrictions, and mandates could be obviated by abandoning the use of "cases" as a metric and focusing on the incidence of serious illness. Early data suggesting increased viral transmission among vaccinated persons, along with the CDC's recent guidance to redon masks for the vaccinated, foreshadow the hopelessness and perpetuity of a case-based strategy to managing the COVID-19 pandemic.

It is possible that no additional safety issues involving the COVID-19 vaccines will arise over time. But, as a factual matter, the answer to this question is unknown today. Stepping beyond voluntary use and moving toward mandates at this early juncture expose organizations and governments to complex risk, and the magnitude of this risk could be tremendous if a significant safety issue is identified in the future. Public health officials have demonstrated time and time again that their ability to accurately predict the future of this pandemic is limited. What is needed from them now is not mandates, but rather honesty and humility, and a focus on preventing serious illness rather than the chimerical goal of preventing cases.

Vaccine Mandates Can't Stop Covid's Spread?[*]
Wall Street Journal, September 16, 2021

Coercion won't work because those without symptoms can still pass on infection.

The Covid-19 pandemic has spurred a remarkable stream of scientific investigation, but that knowledge isn't translating into better public policy. One example is a zealous pursuit of public mask wearing, a measure that has had, at best, a modest effect on viral transmission. Or take lockdowns, shown by research to increase deaths overall but nonetheless still considered an acceptable solution. This intellectual disconnect now extends to Covid-19 vaccine mandates. The policy is promoted as essential for stopping the spread of Covid-19, though the evidence suggests it won't.

Mandates infringe on personal autonomy, which can lead to political strife and unintended consequences, but they have value in some situations. In general, however, wise policy making respects the intrinsic value of personal autonomy and seeks the least burdensome path to achieve social gains.

---

[*] https://www.wsj.com/articles/vaccine-mandate-covid-19-unvaccinated-breakthrough-delta-boosters-fluvoxamine-antibodies-11631820572.

The common argument for vaccine mandates is: You have no right to infect me. But cases are partly driven by asymptomatic and presymptomatic spread—people who are unaware that they even are infected. It isn't practical to punish adults who have no symptoms. This is why other diseases that can be spread by people without symptoms—such as influenza, genital herpes and hepatitis C—are met with policies like voluntary vaccination drives, screening protocols for sexually transmitted diseases, and clean needle exchange programs for intravenous drug users. Doctors and public health officials used to understand that stopping spread is usually not practical.

Here's another problem: The vaccines reduce but don't prevent transmission. Protection from infection appears to wane over time, more noticeably after three to four months, based on a large study of more than 300,000 people in the United Kingdom. As clinical studies from the U.S., Israel, and Qatar show—and many Americans can now personally attest—there is substantial evidence that people who are vaccinated can both contract and contribute to the spread of Covid-19.

This trend has been exacerbated by the Delta variant. The data show that vaccine effectiveness for infection protection fell from roughly 91% to 66% after emergence of the Delta variant, according to a recent CDC report. Data from Israel show rates of protection have declined to less than 40% for some patients. The data still show that people who are vaccinated against Covid-19 are less likely to become infected than people who aren't vaccinated. People who have recovered from Covid-19 appear to have the most protection of all.

But these realities aren't informing vaccine policy. When New York Gov. Kathy Hochul discussed expanding vaccine mandates to state-regulated facilities, she said: "We have to let people know when they walk into our facilities that the people that are taking care of them" are "safe themselves and will not spread this." In fact, the data say they can and will spread it.

The good news is that the vaccines continue to afford significant protection against serious illness from Covid-19. The response from many vaccine advocates has been to promote boosters, and the momentum behind third shots is outpacing the limited data available. The reality is that a more practical approach to managing Covid requires a diverse set of strategies, including using outpatient therapies.

Monoclonal antibodies are still used infrequently, despite evidence showing a substantial risk reduction in hospitalization. The reasons are not well understood but many patients and physicians may be unaware they are available.

There is growing evidence that the antidepressant fluvoxamine is effective, based on the results of a recent, large clinical trial currently undergoing peer review that found a 30% reduction in hospitalization risk. A smaller clinical trial of fluvoxamine published in the Journal of the American Medical Association also found a benefit.

Other medications like hydroxychloroquine and ivermectin, on which health officials seem determined to close the book, are, in reality, unsettled. Controlled clinical trials have yielded conflicting results, but many physicians with substantial experience treating patients with Covid-19—including members of the Early Covid Care Experts group—have reported low rates of hospitalization and death when using these therapies. Some of these patient cohorts are large and have been published in peer-reviewed journals, such as one study of 717 outpatients published in Travel Medicine and Infectious Disease.

Vaccine mandates can't end the spread of the virus as effectiveness declines and new variants emerge. So how can they be a sensible policy? Is it sensible to consign tens of millions of people to an indeterminate number of boosters and the threat of job loss if it isn't clear more doses will stop the spread, either?

The sensible approach, based on the available data, is to promote vaccines for the purpose of preventing serious illness. You

don't need a mandate for this—adults can make their own decisions. But mandates will prolong political conflicts over Covid-19,
and they are an increasingly unsustainable strategy designed to
achieve an unattainable goal.

CHAPTER 12

Making Better Public Health Decisions, Part I

How can leaders do better when the next pandemic threat or public health emergency arrives? How can we in the medical and public health communities avoid the errors of the past? The COVID-19 pandemic demonstrates how important it is to answer these questions.

By almost every important metric, our national policy response to the COVID 19 pandemic was a resounding failure. Americans sacrificed *dearly*, and we have little to show for it. Considering the projected long-term harms from school and university closures, lost opportunities for education and social development of children, and economic injury to small businesses, it is likely that we are worse off now than if public health officials had simply done nothing.

Sadly, much of the scientific community seems resigned to denialism. They see the only failure in public health leadership to be their unwillingness to be even "tougher." Had restrictions only been deeper or more prolonged, they contend, we would have been spared the worst aspects of the pandemic.

But I hope that at least some small proportion of the public health community views the increased distrust of doctors, profound partisanship that has become an integral component of how Americans view public health recommendations, and worsening racial, ethnic, and economic educational disparities brought on by school shutdowns as reasons to honestly reflect on what went wrong and how we can do better.

For those members of the public health community, this chapter is for you. I also want to say that I appreciate your willingness to reexamine the positions you've taken during the pandemic, and your interest in and commitment to bettering the health of the population.

Making Better Decisions

So where should we start? How can we avoid repeating the failed ideas of the past? How do health officials deal with their fear that people will no longer listen to public health recommendations? Or that the public health community will be marginalized? Or that they might lose "control" over a public health crisis, with subsequent unbridled illness or death?

The first step, paradoxically, has nothing to do with the crisis and everything to do with you. The first step is personal improvement. There is nothing more important during a crisis than being the best version of ourselves possible. This is because of how crises challenge us both personally and professionally. The former is most important because it affects how we show up for the latter. I will discuss the latter first.

Professionally, the challenges of a crisis demand that we apply our intellectual and creative resources, our collaborative talents, and our endurance. This is a challenge for everyone and, in a way, defines what it means to be in a crisis situation. A crisis can push us to extremes of our performance and redefine the boundaries of our scope of responsibilities. All of this, of course, is a perfect recipe for pushing our buttons on a personal level, which is why personal improvement is central to powerful leadership.

On a *personal* level, crises magnify our self-doubt, concerns, and fears. It's almost uncanny how similar questions arise for each of us in the face of a crisis. What if I am not competent enough? What if I am not smart enough? What if I make the wrong decision? What if I am blamed for a poor outcome? How do I deal with a political or business leader whose cooperation I need, but whose views and interests are completely unaligned with mine? What if people hate me, laugh at me, ridicule me, or dismiss me?

And then on an even deeper personal level, do any of us really believe our performance at work is not affected by the quality of the relationships we have with our spouse, children, parents, relatives, and friends? The successes and challenges of those relationships spill out onto our professional performance, and vice versa.

All together, these are the reasons that personal improvement is the most important first step to take if a leader's goal is to maximize his or her likelihood of achieving favorable outcomes during a crisis. You cannot lead with maximum effectiveness if your thinking is not clear, and you can't achieve clarity without first doing some internal housecleaning.

Based on my own experience working with Christopher Maher, the direction my life has taken both before and after this experience, and my observations of health officials and political leaders during the pandemic, my humble opinion is that fear is the most important emotion to investigate, to explore to its deepest roots, and to (hopefully) become free of. Fear is pervasive in our society, can be found at the center of most—if not all—social and political conflicts, and is second only to love in its power and ability to move hearts and minds.

My experience has taught me that the journey toward personal improvement is at least as important as the destination for two reasons: first, there is no way to reach the destination of being free from fear without setting out on the journey; and second, setting out on the journey activates providence, and heavenly forces join us along our path. By "providence," I mean those heavenly forces—angels, spirits, and other universal entities—that shape the direction our lives take and help clear a path toward the lessons we are intended to learn.

As a public health leader, the benefit of being as free as possible from fear may be best understood by considering how deeply embedded it is in every layer of our existence. For me, it permeated *everything*, from how I walked, how I laughed, how much pain or tightness I felt in different joints and muscles, the thoughts that sprang into my mind, and every single aspect of how I related to other human beings—and not for the better. The presence of fear makes it impossible to access the parts of our brains and beings that are active when we feel peace, joy, gratitude, or happiness.

Who would ever opt to enter a crisis situation without access to his or her full capacity? No one who wants to be as effective and successful as possible. Yet, a fearful consciousness characterizes America's public health response to COVID-19.

The Journey to Freedom

There are different pathways to getting free from fear, and my personal belief is that each individual has his or her own unique path and journey. The guidance for how to set out on this journey can either come from your own God-given intuition, if you are so blessed, or the intuition of those around you who are more connected to the spiritual realm. I would put myself in the latter category, and God kindly brought me a wife and partner who was in the former. Brianna has been my spiritual guide, and I would not be where I am today without her. Period.

Why is the journey worthwhile? Because it will create new realities that are impossible to achieve—or even conceive of—otherwise. For me, if I had not set out on my own journey of personal improvement, I would not have been able to publish editorials in the *Wall Street Journal* with clarity that was uncommon at the time or serve today as Florida's state surgeon general. It may be helpful to recognize that the most challenging scenarios—those that arouse our fears, anxieties, and desires—are impossible to navigate in ways that align with our values without first exorcising the inner gremlins.

Sometimes, people ask me how I knew the things I did so early in the pandemic, particularly ideas that were considered unorthodox or incorrect at the time, but then became more widely embraced as time went on. These ideas include my certainty that lockdowns would achieve very little, my belief that school shutdowns would ultimately harm kids, my doubts that mask mandates would have any substantial effect on the pandemic, and my skepticism about the practicality and morality of COVID-19 vaccine passports.

I had no special training per se. After all, there are countless physicians in the United States with backgrounds in public health and research science. I also had no special professional experience per se. I was only about a decade out of medical school and residency training when the pandemic started.

What I did have, however, was a mind largely free of the temptations that arise during crises, like fear and panic. That made it infinitely easier to see facts and events for what they truly were—rather than the boogeymen they were made out to be when viewed through the lens of fear and panic—and learn what I needed from these data in order to arrive at the best policy proposals possible.

Countless books, courses, and programs have been developed for personal improvement, and people have reported various degrees of success with them. As long as a program resonates with you, and you have no indication that the program has ill intentions (unfortunately, some organizations prey on other people's aspirations to better themselves and the world), I think it's more important to act decisively and move forward rather than agonizing over picking the "perfect" program. Plus, as earlier discussed, the moment you undertake a journey of genuine self-improvement, providence will be on your side.

Imagine how the last two years would have gone if public health leadership in the United States had rejected fear, embraced reality about the limitations inherent in stopping the spread of a contagious respiratory virus, and respected the autonomy of each human being to make decisions about things like whether to leave their family business open, attend school in-person, or receive a new vaccine?

We would have suffered none of the flip-flopping or political grandstanding that characterized the pandemic, such as the musical chairs performance of public health guidance that started with no masks (Dr. Fauci in March 2020), then changed to cloth masks, then changed to double masking, then changed to surgical masks, and currently stands as a hodgepodge of nuanced, but equally unsupported, positions. A similar pattern unfolded for COVID-19 vaccine mandates, which evolved from no mandates (as President Biden promised Americans in December

2020), to mandates for certain activities, to mandates for certain populations, to mandates for virtually everyone, and is now a confused mishmash of vaccine mandate policies.

In this same imaginary scenario, schools would have remained open, small businesses and gyms would not have been forced to close, and health officials would have avoided mandates that primarily served to stir acrimony without providing any substantial health benefits. These outcomes are the inevitable result of mindful public health leadership.

While we don't know what public health crisis lies next around the corner, we do know it is coming. Leaders who remain servants to their inner fears, anxieties, and desires will never be able to serve the public as powerfully as they otherwise could. For those public health leaders who want to do better next time, I hope you choose to either start or continue your journey to freedom.

CHAPTER 13

Making Better Public Health Decisions, Part II

In the last chapter, I discussed how pursuing personal improvement is the first and most important step leaders should take in order to make better public health decisions. The second step is to pursue training in the field of decision science. While I was in graduate school at Harvard, I took several courses in decision science, a critically important discipline that can substantially reduce the odds of public health leaders making errors as egregious as those we have seen over the past two-and-a-half years. I was required to attain a certain level of expertise because I was in a doctoral program, but an introductory course is probably sufficient for most in public health leadership positions.

The Center for Health Decision Science at the Harvard T.H. Chan School of Public Health defines decision science as "the collection of quantitative techniques used to inform decision-making at the individual and population levels . . . . It includes decision analysis, risk analysis, cost-benefit and cost-effectiveness analysis, constrained optimization, simulation modeling, and behavioral decision theory, as well as parts of operations research, microeconomics, statistical inference, management control, cognitive and social psychology, and computer science." They go on further to say that "decision science provides a unique framework for understanding public health problems, and for improving policies to address those problems."

What this unwieldy mouthful essentially means is that that decision science is a mathematical approach to analyzing decisions (both large and small) that incorporates information about risks, trade-offs, values, and preferences. The method is particularly useful when an individual, such as a health official or policymaker, has to make a decision but has multiple options that represent different risks and trade-offs. Because it uses a mathematical framework, decision science is both transparent and reproducible.

The advantage of incorporating decision science when facing public health problems is that it forces decision-makers to be explicit about what factors are important to a decision and transparent in their approach to addressing a problem. This means being explicit about the options, the anticipated consequences associated with those options, and the value of the different outcomes. For these reasons, applying the methods of decision science is perhaps most needed when public health challenges are complex.

The power of decision science for policymakers and public health leaders is that it crowds out the possibility of magical thinking—something we saw often during the pandemic—and can often protect an individual from making overtly poor decisions.

School closures are a good example of how valuable decision analysis can be. In the decision over whether to close schools, a very basic analysis—one that many Americans just did intuitively—would have shown that closing schools was an enormously costly decision with little upside. This would have been clear by considering the enormous beneficial effects that education, consistency in life routines, and social support bear on the health of children, and the data that already demonstrated the extraordinarily low risk that COVID-19 posed to children.

These data would have dictated that the analytically "correct" course of action would be to avoid closures, since only a highly beneficial intervention with a high certainty of success could justify closing schools. Even then, one would almost certainly want the closures to be brief.

Let me say this in a different way. It would have been *impossible* for any public health official, academic researcher, or policy analyst with training in decision sciences to conclude that the health benefits of prolonged school closures outweighed their risks. The best available data showed that schools were not substantially contributing to spread, and the harms associated with prolonged school closures were inferable from decades of research on the value of childhood education. Irrespective of a person's political allegiance, there could only be one valid conclusion.

Because decision analysis is a mathematical approach and almost always requires making some assumptions, there is, of course, an opportunity for dishonest individuals to put a thumb on the scale in order to skew results. But some issues are so black-and-white—including the obvious harms from prolonged school closures—that no degree of subtle mathematical maneuvering could possibly change the outcome. If public health officials were required to support their recommendations using decision science, it would have prevented much of the equivocating and grandstanding that ultimately hurt America's children.

Decision science could also have been used to compare the value of different COVID-19 testing strategies. Undoubtedly, such an analysis would have demonstrated that the value of testing low-risk people or people without symptoms was lower than the value of testing high-risk people or people with symptoms. This is because most transmission happens early in the disease course anyway—often before COVID-19 testing is performed—and most harm is concentrated in people who are high risk. Therefore, excessive testing strategies among the asymptomatic or among colleges students, for example, were bound to be a low-value proposition.

In addition, decision sciences can help us avoid economic waste. While COVID-19 test manufacturers were surely pleased about school district decisions to implement routine "surveillance" testing, this low-value exercise wasted vast sums that could undoubtedly have been used for much more valuable public health activities, such as smoking cessation programs or physical activity promotion. Similarly, it is difficult to imagine the quantity of resources that were wasted by millions of asymptomatic international travelers who chased after pretravel COVID-19 tests so they could return to their home countries.

Courses in decision sciences are offered at universities around the country with established research programs in health policy, such as the University of Michigan, the University of Minnesota, Harvard, and Stanford. Some universities may also offer remote learning programs, which eliminates one potential hurdle to enrollment and engagement. Good textbooks for the public health community have also been published, and these may be perfect for the self-learner. One example is *Decision Making in Health and Medicine* by Dr. M. G. Myriam Hunink, but a favorite of mine that is out of print but still available used is *Clinical Decision Analysis* by Dr. Milton Weinstein.

Based on the abysmal performance of public health officials over the past two-and-a-half years, it is reasonable to strongly encourage—if not require—this type of training for influential public health officials. But as powerful a tool as decision science is for public health policymaking, it will never reach its potential unless it is in the hands of mindful leaders. Decision analysis is no substitute for mindful leadership, and pursuing personal improvement remains important. Why? Because it is one thing to know what the right thing to do is, but another thing to actually do it.

The former may require decision science to determine, but the latter requires clear and fearless leadership to execute. Moreover, some problems are too complex or the unknowns too great to place any confidence in mathematical models, and at the end of the day, there is no substitute for human ingenuity.

Public health officials who want to be prepared for the next emergency should complete training in decision science. It only requires time, discipline, and a commitment to serving the public as powerfully as possible.

CHAPTER 14

Fear versus Freedom

Freedom is a value that was often dismissed during the COVID-19 pandemic, but I pray that its importance is not forgotten in future health crises. It was a casualty because of its direct relationship with fear; where one exists, the other cannot.

What I mean by that is the "price" of fear is that it robs us of our ability to emotionally and spiritually connect with other people. The "payoff" of freedom is that it nurtures and facilitates that same emotional and spiritual connection. And that emotional and spiritual connection also serves to grow our appreciation of freedom, since freedom is intrinsic to our souls as human beings. The cycle is virtuous.

Public health leaders who are as free as possible from fear and have undertaken the journey to achieve freedom from their own inner challenges are those in whom we can place the most trust. Those individuals will make the best public health decisions. By virtue of who they are and what they value, they are the most likely to tackle problems from an expansive perspective while still respecting individual sovereignty to the extent possible. The value of these individuals is even more pronounced during a crisis, when the temptation to circumvent individual sovereignty in pursuit of a "solution" is greatest.

Measures that severely restrict a person's freedom should only be used in emergent situations, and always with the greatest degree of caution. In a hospital setting, for example, when a patient is extremely agitated and concern arises about risk of harm to self or others, there are steps doctors can take to control the situation. The most severe of these are physical restraints, for which there are very specific rules regulating how often the patient must be reevaluated, for the obvious reason that it is inhumane to keep someone restrained for any longer than is absolutely necessary. The same model should be applied to the implementation of the severest public health measures.

The argument that "your freedom to swing your fist ends just where my nose begins" is often cited as a rationale for subverting individual sovereignty in public health affairs. But invocation of this as some immutable law or maxim is either lazy thinking or rationalization in pursuit of an end.

This old maxim has very limited utility, because in public health, the effects that our actions have on the health of others fall on a spectrum. On one end are actions that have no effect on the health of other people. For example, if I were to eat a pint of ice cream pumped full of harmful artificial ingredients alone in the privacy of my own home, that action, in general, will have no immediate effect on the health of other people. On the other hand, if I were to be diagnosed with active tuberculosis and then walk around a restaurant coughing on people, that choice is likely to impose immediate harm to the health of many other people.

Whereas the former should be met with education and possibly other measures to reduce consumption of junk food, the latter ought to be met with restrictions and prohibitions. These restrictions and prohibitions might even require legal enforcement. Everything else is in between, and that in-between area captures a slew of health states and behaviors.

We may walk around and unknowingly spread germs to others. Our choices to eat healthily or unhealthily may inadvertently influence the dietary decisions of friends and neighbors who observe us. Our choice of vehicle may affect the quality of air in our neighborhood. In other words, sometimes our fists don't touch the noses of other people, sometimes it's a glancing blow, and sometimes it's a full-on whomp, but no one who participates in society is entitled to absolute freedom from having their nose bruised now and then. As human beings living together in a society, there's no practical way around it.

The role of leaders is to find the right balance, the right set point along the spectrum. There is no formula for this. Each scenario has to be evaluated thoughtfully.

During the pandemic, for example, individuals who demanded that others around them wear masks were asking for something that was not well matched to where that health behavior fell along the spectrum. Considering how personal and private a personal's face is, the long history of randomized clinical trials that had failed to show a substantial benefit from wearing masks, and the strong aversion that many felt toward the practice, a wise leader would never have tried to implement this policy.

As I said earlier, there is no formula for this type of decision making. Decision science helps, and cleaning house emotionally and spiritually helps even more. Combined, these approaches have the best chance of producing mindful leadership that is best equipped to help the public navigate future health challenges and crises.

I will end this book with a note about Governor Ron DeSantis, who exemplifies mindful leadership. The world is blessed to have him, and his current position as governor of Florida in this moment of history is a representation of God's providence. During a period of profound darkness, he has carried the torch of light and freedom, with an authenticity and integrity that no other leader possesses. He is also blessed with humility and a genuine commitment to doing what he believes is the right thing to do. I am proud and honored to fight alongside him, because humanity is worth it one million times over.

Afterword

By Gavin de Becker

Throughout world history, people in power have used fear to influence and control populations—fear of outside invaders that don't ever invade, fear of demons and devils that can't be seen, fear of terrorism that might happen but hasn't, fear of earthquakes that never come, and, of course, fear of communicable diseases.

Because fear works so well, leaders and governments are expert at crafting enemies that only they can protect you from. The most useful enemies are flexible: they can change and evolve, so they keep their currency. Promoting fear of an actual enemy, like Russia in the 1950s, eventually has limitations because the enemy is real, with real features we can see. That's why those in power switched from fear of Russia to promoting fear of communists, then switched to communism, an ideology.

Over time, the things we are told to fear become harder for regular citizens to see for themselves. First, it's countries that sponsor terrorists, then unseen terrorists who might be conspiring to kill us, then terrorism itself. And a war on terror can never end, for there is no beachhead to capture—there's no consistent *there* there. This kind of war needs very little maintenance, just the occasional scary story about a terror plot, easy to identify (when real), and easy to conjure anytime, since those in power are the ones deciding who will be branded as a terrorist, and what qualifies as terrorism. Enemies of the State are always identified by the State, which also decides how credible a threat is, what information the citizens can know, and how the story of each near-miss terrorist plot will be presented to us.

I know this all sounds cynical, but be patient, it gets worse. The things we are told to fear become smaller and more diffuse, until they are invisible. The village witch doctor maintained his power because he was the only one who could see the evil spirit that had entered your soul—and only he could chase away the invisible danger with strings of beads or mystical incantations. Today, we are told to fear a sneaky microscopic asymptomatic virus that sometimes can be seen only by a test.

Before 2020, going backward through time for centuries, the presence of problematic symptoms was the obvious defining factor for determining someone had a disease. Not so nowadays, when people can be ordered into isolation because of a test result, a result that doesn't mean you're about to get sick (most aren't) and doesn't mean you can make anyone else sick (most can't).

The viral particle has thus become history's most useful object of fear: impossible to see, impossible to stop, could be hiding in anyone, could already be inside you, government controls the data, and best of all, a virus mutates into new viruses we are told to fear. It's a goose that keeps laying golden eggs, golden for those in power, producing unending scary warnings, death counts on the news, lockdowns, mandates, and doctors telling us about the ever-evolving danger.

In this context, we meet Dr. Joe Ladapo, a public health official who doesn't want to scare you, a doctor who consciously *avoids* frightening people. Imagine that. He expresses accurate information, cares about fairness, cares about people, uses objectivity, science, experience, and training—and doesn't use fear.

Since 2020, in the name of your safety, the federal government has been willing to change all the rules and knock down all the guardrails. Anything goes. But not for Dr. Ladapo. In a time when public health dehumanizes the individual, Dr. Ladapo remembers that the public is made up of individuals, people worth caring about. Imagine that.

Yet some Americans love to have their fears, and for a while, many loved to listen to the reliable voice of Anthony Fauci, reliable in that he always ends on something scary, every summary including *could, perhaps, might, concerning, substantial, worth watching closely, uptick in the numbers.*

I'm often asked what we should fear, but there is no *should* involved, because true fear is not voluntary. It will come and get your attention when needed, whether you want it to or not. Conversely, most worrying is voluntary. To understand all this, we must start with the odd ways people evaluate risk. There are Americans who'd never visit a place like Egypt for fear of being killed there, so they stay home, where the risk of murder is twenty times greater. Though smoking kills more people in an afternoon than lightning does in a year, there are those who calm their fear during a lightning storm by . . . smoking a cigarette. On their way to the airport, people afraid of flying obsess about an air crash while doing one of the riskiest things Americans ever do: driving without paying attention. (Do you imagine the jumbo jet captain is distracted from piloting by the fear of car accidents? I hope not, though that concern would be statistically more valid.)

Unlike true fear, unwarranted fear is rarely logical. I met a woman who feared she might have contracted the "flesh-eating" disease that she had seen on the news. (It crossed my mind that she could have told me this before shaking my hand, but no matter.) She didn't have the flesh-eating disease or mad cow disease, nor is she likely to die in an earthquake or a jet crash. But a little worry never hurt anybody, right? Wrong.

Anxiety kills more Americans each year than all the dangers named above (through high blood pressure, heart disease, immunosuppression, depression, and a myriad of other stress-related ailments). Fear is often more harmful than the outcomes we dread. It just might be that thirty years of fearing skin cancer detracts more quality from one's life than three weeks of managing the medical crisis and moving on.

Worry is the fear we manufacture, and those who choose to do it certainly have a wide range of dangers to dwell upon. Television stations in most major cities produce up to forty hours a day of original programming telling us about those who have fallen prey to some disaster and exploring what calamities may be coming next. The local news anchor should begin each evening's broadcast by saying, "Welcome to the news; we're surprised you made it through another day. Here's what happened to those who didn't."

Among all the dangers, the clever virus is the hardest to dodge. Turns out nothing can reliably keep it out of our noses. More important, it seems nothing can keep it out of our minds, which is not surprising given that the most powerful institutions in history—the US government, corporate media, and Pharma—are investing billions to scare people into submission. The pharmaceutical product they are pushing (and pushing hard) is now the most widely ingested consumer product in history. If the powers that be have their way, it will be consumed by every person on Earth. Ambitious, bold, impressive, and scary.

Yet here's the thing: It isn't COVID we need to learn to live with; it's life itself we need to learn to live with. Life: sexually transmitted, incurable, and always fatal. Life, with all its risks and uncertainties.

For two years and counting, federal public health officials have focused on just one risk: COVID-19, as if the rest of reality would pull over and wait by the side of the road, wait for Anthony Fauci's motorcade to pass. But it won't pass; it just keeps getting longer, and slower, congesting the flow of traffic that used to let us get home each day, to rest, and to live our lives. Anytime those in power focus on just one thing, they are acting against Nature, which, you'll recall, is comprised of many things that interact to create and sustain life.

Here's a thought experiment: What would you want in a personal physician? Would you want a doctor who intentionally scares you, restricts your freedom, believes that controlling you will control a virus—and keeps believing that even after all his measures fail. After you do exactly what the doctor told you to do, you keep finding yourself back in the waiting room with COVID—again. Double vaccinated and double boosted, and back in the waiting room with COVID—again. Wearing two masks, yet back in the waiting room again.

As you saw in these pages, Dr. Joe Ladapo is a man willing to share his humanity with you, a man who remembers that the health of the public is not reached through suppression and control, but through compassion and care. Aren't those the characteristics you'd want in your personal physician?

And wouldn't you welcome a public health official who believes this:

Measures that severely restrict a person's freedom should only be used in emergent situations, and always with the greatest degree of caution. In a hospital setting, for example, when a patient is extremely agitated and concern arises about risk of harm to self or others, there are steps doctors can take to control the situation. The most severe of these are physical restraints, for which there are very specific rules regulating how often the patient must be reevaluated, for the obvious reason that it is inhumane to keep someone restrained for any longer than is absolutely necessary. The same model should be applied to the implementation of the severest public health measures.

The fortunate citizens of Florida have just such a physician helping them decide what's best for them—and by "them," I mean each individual. If you're enjoying the freedom and medical moderation in Florida today, it's not just luck; it's also Joe Ladapo. For the rest of the country, he's created a model of how it would be if the attributes any of us would want in a personal physician resided in our public health officials.

Thank you, Joe, for sharing who you are with us, for honoring who we are, and for knowing that freedom and accurate information are good for our health.

—Gavin de Becker, bestselling author of *The Gift of Fear*